ROCKyourBODY™

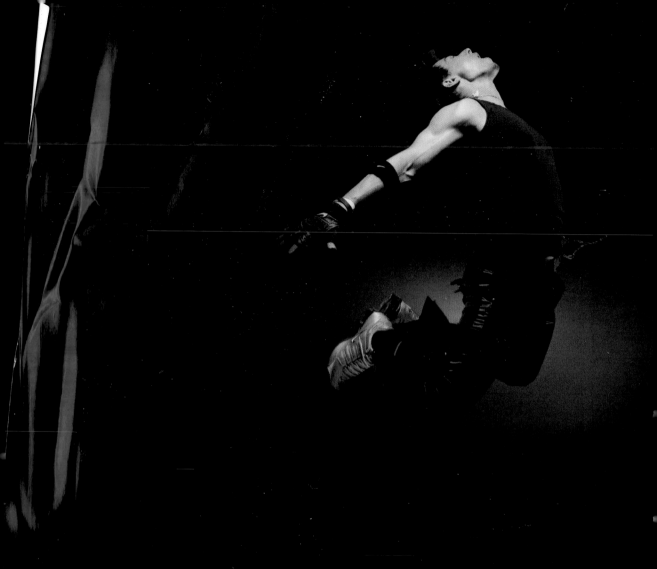

There's no such thing as a bad dancer.
Dance is **personal**. Dance is **spiritual.**
Dance belongs to the **individual.**
Only the individual can judge.

ROCK your BODY™

THE **ULTIMATE HIP-HOP INSPIRED WORKOUT** TO **SLIM, SHAPE,** AND **STRENGTHEN YOUR BODY**

JAMIE KING

celebrity director/choreographer and creator of the Nike Rockstar Workout

RODALE

Rodale books may be purchased for business or promotional use or for special sales. For information, please write to: Special Markets Department, Rodale Inc., 733 Third Avenue, New York, NY 10017

Printed in the United States of America

Rodale Inc. makes every effort to use acid-free ∞, recycled paper ♻.

Cover and interior book design by Chris Rhoads

Photo editor: Marc Sirinsky

Celebrity photographs have been provided courtesy of the individual celebrities except where otherwise noted. The photographs appearing on pages 30 and 46 are courtesy of Daniel Sladek. The photograph appearing on page 72 is courtesy of Nike. Exercise photographs © Joan Allen

"Nike Rockstar Workout" is a trademark of Nike, Inc.
"Rock Your Body" is a trademark of King Productions, Inc.

Executive producer/management: Daniel Sladek; producer/choreographer: Tabitha Dumo; associate producer/choreographer: Carla Kama; assistant choreographer: Alyson Faulk; production coordinator: Candice Coke; rehearsal video coordinator: Walid Azami; assistants to Jamie King: Kelly Ann Anthony and Sasha Boni; music producer: DJ Backdraft; legal representation: William Skrzyniarz, Esq., and Glenn Litwak, Esq.; agency representation: Creative Artists Agency, Trident Media Group, and McDonald Selznick & Associates

Library of Congress Cataloging-in-Publication Data

King, Jamie.
    Rock your body : the ultimate hip-hop inspired workout to slim, shape, and strengthen your body / Jamie King.
        p.   cm.
    Includes index.
    ISBN–13 978–1–59486–566–4   paperback
    ISBN–10 1–59486–566–3   paperback
    1. Aerobic dancing.   2. Hip-hop dance.   I. Title.
    RA781.15.K56   2007
    613.7'15—dc22   2007005845

Distributed to the trade by Holtzbrinck Publishers

2 4 6 8 10 9 7 5 3 1   paperback

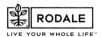

We inspire and enable people to improve their lives and the world around them

For more of our products visit **rodalestore.com** or call 800-848-4735

For my **parents**

—**J.K.**

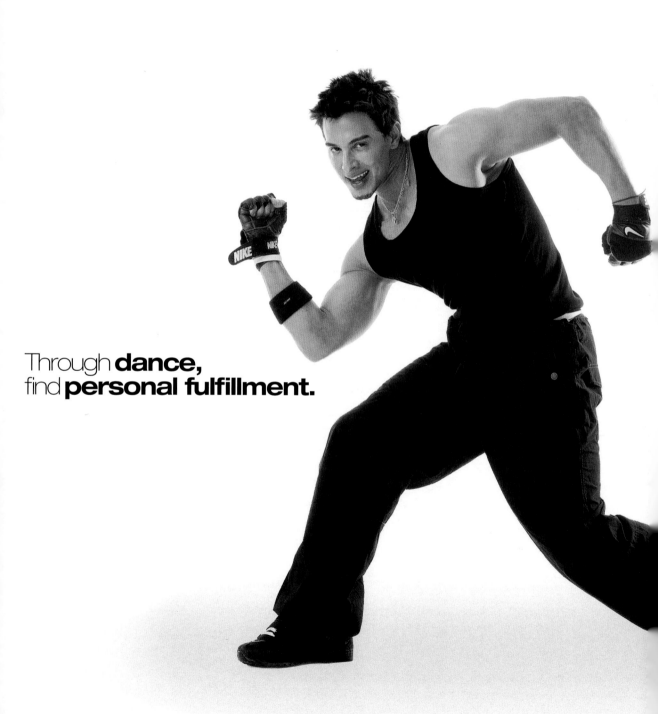

Through **dance,**
find **personal fulfillment.**

Contents

Part I: Rock Your Mind, Body, and Soul

Part II: Rock Your Body Workout

Part III: Rock Your Diet

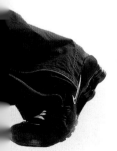

Acknowledgments

Seeing *Rock Your Body* come to fruition has been an enormous pleasure because it's given me the opportunity to share the joy of dance. But this project would not have been possible without the help and encouragement of my extraordinarily loving, supportive, and talented family, friends, and colleagues.

They include, first and foremost, my family—my mom, Barbara Watts, who gave me the gift of groove. As a single mother, she did a fantastic job under difficult circumstances and made me feel special, which boosted my confidence so I could pursue my dreams. I also want to thank my stepfather, David, who forced me to study. Because he insisted that I work hard in school, I had to work even harder to keep dance in my life. He also instilled in me the spirit of dance.

I want to thank my Aunt Patti, who gave me the soul of dance. When babysitting me, she used to dance in her living room to old R&B songs and encouraged me to express myself in movement. Soon I was trying to gain the spotlight by making up my own dances for family and friends. Her passion was contagious.

My grandmother, Lois Barker, still dances in her retirement community in Arizona. Having her as my grandmother allowed me to understand that joy can be found in dance at any age. She still inspires me. I love you.

I also want to express my thanks to my dance teacher, Sharon Butler, who believed in me from the very beginning and helped me believe in myself. She encouraged me to pursue a career in dance and even accompanied me to the dance convention where I made my first contacts in the professional dance world. I met Joe Tremaine at that convention, and he gave me a scholarship to his terrific school in Los Angeles. For that and many other things, I thank Joe.

I also drew inspiration from the director-choreographer Debbie Allen, the television series *Fame* (I totally identified with the hero Leroy, who never gave up, no matter what), and MTV for its amazing introduction to pop culture. I learned so much from watching Michael Jackson and Janet Jackson, Prince and Madonna. I had their posters pinned up all over my room. Their careers showed me what was possible when you follow your passion.

Gene Kelly inspired me because he was an athletic dancer. I watched him in old movie clips. He was masculine when he danced, yet he had such grace. He proved that dance and sport belong together just as much as art and dance. It's what got me to this place.

I also have been helped by my spiritual advisor, Marcus Weston, an instructor at the Kabbalah Center, who taught me how to truly dance through life, and Rav and Karen Berg, who encourage me to never stop sharing my gift and all its benefits with the world.

I thank my support team, my manager, Daniel Sladek, and my agents, Tony Selznick and Julie McDonald, who back me up in whatever complicated scenario I devise, either onstage or on the page. This book and the *Rock Your Body* DVD would not have been possible without the dedication of my lawyer William Skrzyniarz, CAA's Adam Devajian, and agent Eileen Cope of the Trident Media Group, who kept the faith. And a special thanks to nutritionist Debra Wein, MS, RD, for her help on the nutritional side of rocking your body.

I also depend on my angels in my personal life and at King Productions: Derek Loura (thank you, D), Tabitha Dumo (you rock), Kelly Ann Anthony, Sasha Boni, my sis Candice Coke, Kristen Hetland, Naomi Priestly, Stef Roos, and Tiff Olsen. Without their patience and support, I couldn't extend myself in so many directions.

Nike greatly facilitated my getting out the message that "dance is sport," my credo. It gave me a fantastic platform from which to spread my enthusiasm for dance around the world.

A big thank-you to my editor Zach Schisgal, Joan Allen, Andrew Gelman, Chris Rhoads, Liz Perl, Gunnar Waldman, Ron Fried, Beth Mayerowitz, Nancy N. Bailey, Cathy Pawlowski, Marc Sirinsky, and the entire team at Rodale. Thanks also to the Showdown Productions team for making my Rock Your Body DVD a success, and to Debra Gordon for your tremendous contribution.

I sincerely appreciate the contributions made by Madonna, Christina Aguilera, Mari Winsor, Miss Prissy, Mia Michaels, Carmen Electra, Laurie Ann Gibson, Rihanna, Carrie Ann Inaba, Ricky Martin, Toni Basil, Omar Lopez, Joe Tremaine, Robin Antin, Tracy Gray, Stacey Stafford, Carmit Bacher, Matthew Rolston, Julie Daugherty, Mariah Carey, Pink, Britney Spears, Rain, Jeri Slaughter, Darcy Winslow, Kenny Ortega, Tyra Banks, Omar Cruz, Jeff Margolis, Richmond and Tone Talauega, Rasta Thomas, Kelly Perkins, Debra Wein, Angela Becker, Brian Graden, Benny Medina, Steven Klein, Carlos Serrao, Dave Hogan, Chris Taaffe, Guy Oseary, Glenn Campbell, Jim DeYonkers, Markus Klinko and Indrani, Ellen Von Unwerth, and their respective agents, managers, and publicists.

Finally, I want to thank anyone who's ever shared the love of dance and the desire to dance, and anyone who has ever expressed themselves through movement. This book is for you!

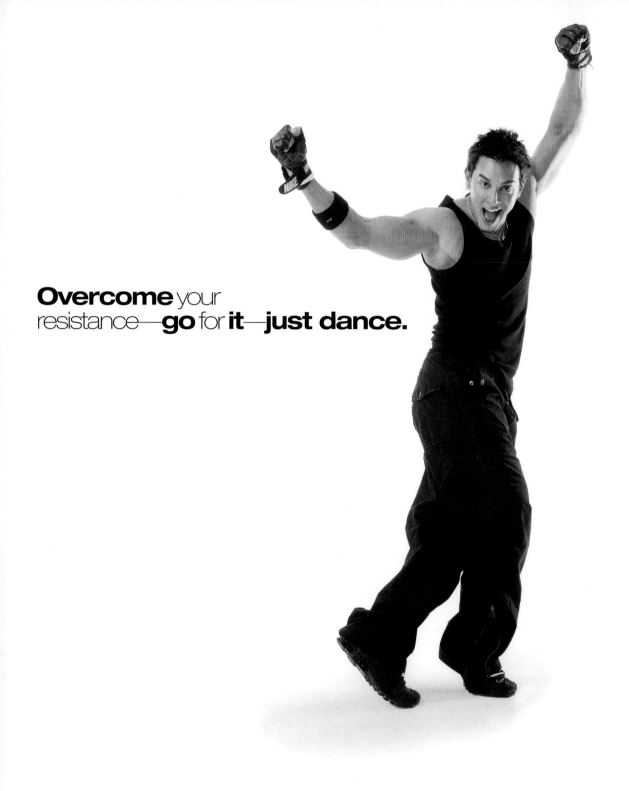

Overcome your resistance—**go** for **it**—just dance.

Introduction

A lot of people have been asking me why I've written this book—especially during a year in which I was also directing Madonna's record-shattering *Confessions* world tour as well as her hit music video "Sorry," Asian superstar Rain's world tour, Christina Aguilera's *Back to Basics* world tour, Mariah Carey and Shakira's live performances on the MTV Video Music Awards broadcast, and last, but certainly not least, directing Ricky Martin's *Black and White* tour! Not to mention my ongoing work with Nike! Because I'm crazy, I guess . . . No, just kidding. Actually, I wrote this book to share my gift of dance with the world and to infect people everywhere with the spirit of dance—no matter what their body type, background, or history.

Listen, I'm not a doctor, I'm not a trainer, I'm not a nutritionist or physical therapist. What I am is a lifelong dancer.

I feel like I was given this amazing gift of dance and movement and expression. Now I want to pass that gift on to you. Because I'm more than just a dancer; I'm an artist and a creator. My job is to teach people how to express themselves through dance. And I don't care if you're a rock star or a lawyer—I want to teach *you*.

There's another reason I've written this book, however, one that plays into my own reasons for doing the work I do: to make you happy. I know, I know . . . that sounds kind of cheesy. But the reality is that dancing, whether you're doing it yourself or watching others, just makes you feel *good*. Listen to the music, watch the movement, and before you know it your own foot starts tapping to the beat, a grin breaks out on your face, and your body begins moving on its own.

To me, there is nothing more life affirming than dance. I started as a kid in my living room in the small town of Verona, Wisconsin, dancing to videos on MTV. My inspiration? Debbie Allen, who starred in the hit television show *Fame*. I first learned about dance from watching that show, and she defined for me everything a choreographer is and should be.

Growing up, plenty of people told me that I couldn't succeed. But I refused to believe them. I overcame their negativity by realizing that I could be whom I wanted to be if I just stayed focused and believed in myself. My inner determination helped, but dance itself also helped.

Today I'm known as the "go to" dance/music/performance director. From Madonna to Ricky Martin, from Jennifer Lopez to Christina Aguilera, I'm the one behind the scenes, creating the visions you see onstage and on the screen. My goal is to break boundaries, move beyond the expected, pull things out of my rock stars even *they* didn't know they had. That's why, I think, I've been so successful in this game of life. I like to encourage, not discourage.

I could continue on in this vein, working only with the rich and famous, but I've always been passionate about bringing this gift of dance to a larger audience. While I love working with celebrities, I also love working with people who aren't in show business: teenagers, young mothers, athletes, students, and office workers. People like you, who don't yet understand how thrilling and entertaining it is to use dance to stay fit, and how dance can revolutionize your life.

I finally got my chance in 2004 when Nike asked me to become its global spokesperson for dance fitness. I created the Nike Rockstar Workout, proving to the world that dance is an intense fitness program, not just something nice to watch. Since then, the Nike Rockstar Workout has been performed at hundreds of conventions and media events around the world. It's offered at gyms around the globe. And it has given me an incredible opportunity to spread my belief that dance can change your life.

Still it wasn't enough. There were still millions of people out there, I knew, who were scared of dance, certain they couldn't do it, convinced that dance wasn't really a "workout," that it was something only for the stars. What they—what *you*—don't realize is that through dance, *everyone* is a star.

And so *Rock Your Body* was born.

Throughout this book (and the *Rock Your Body* DVD, which you can purchase in stores and online at www.rockyourbodyprogram.com), you'll learn how to unleash your inner dancer and bring dance into your everyday life. You'll also learn why dance is one of the best fitness workouts you'll ever do, and why it is so much more than just a way to get in shape physically—it's also a way to get in shape emotionally.

Through the Rock Your Body program, you'll learn how to be as fit as Madonna and as sexy as Rihanna. You'll learn how to move like Ricky Martin and tone your body like Britney Spears. You know why? Because I'm the guy who teaches them how to move like that! Now I've taken that training, those regimens, those dance steps, together with my own personal mantras, and brought them to you as my gift.

Many workouts have been published over the past few years, but what makes *Rock Your Body* different is that I introduce hot dance steps that have been featured in the latest music videos and concert tours. These moves tone every part of your body, increase your flexibility and strength, and promote weight loss—and they give you sexy moves to use on the dance floor. Forget "no pain, no gain" fitness routines; dancing isn't just work, it's fun, creative, and physically challenging . . . and boy do I love a challenge.

My team and I worked as hard to develop the Rock Your Body workout as we've worked on any performance. We spent months coming up with entertaining dance sequences to challenge you physically while boosting you emotionally. We made sure to develop moves you could easily follow. Plus, the photographs in this book show you exactly how to twist your body, lift your legs, roll your shoulders, and complete a hundred other moves to obtain the full benefits of the Rock Your Body workout. Don't worry—I'll be with you the whole way through—just pay attention to the photos!

As you read this book, I want you to keep thinking, "Yes, I can do this. I can become fit, hip, and get moving. I can be a rock star!" Because the bottom line is that it's possible for anyone to dance.

While the voice you hear in the book is primarily mine, you'll also hear from many people I work with—rock stars like Madonna, Rain, and Pink—and fellow choreographers and directors like Kenny Ortega, Laurie Ann Gibson, and the Talauega brothers. Some of them you know, some of them you've never heard of, but I've chosen them to speak out in my book because of their influence on their craft and their strong feelings about dance. Listen to what they have to say about dance, about me, about their perspective on life: Their lessons are worth learning.

To provide a holistic, comprehensive tune-up for your body and life, I also worked with Debra Wein, MS, RD, the nutritionist for the Boston Ballet, to create the Dancer's Diet—a new way of eating designed to make you healthier and more energetic.

By the time you've integrated the Rock Your Body program into your daily life—nutrition as well as dance—you'll not only be fitter and feel better, but you'll have entered a new dimension in your life, one where mind, body, and spirit converge. You'll have entered the magical world of dance. Your rewards will be physical, emotional, and even spiritual. Most of all, don't be afraid to dance. Just do it!

www.jamiekingofficial.com

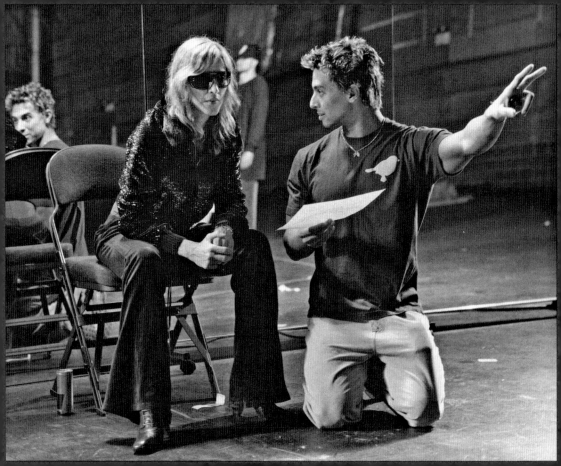

Madonna

JAMIE ON MADONNA: I directed Madonna's *Confessions, Re-Invention,* and *Drowned World* world tours, and her "Sorry" music video. She is a perfect example of how dance can keep you fit and in shape and looking beautiful. She is both the ultimate showgirl and the ultimate businesswoman. She ran off and became the biggest female star in history. She's influenced the world. She really epitomizes the American Dream. But to do what she's done she had to have incredible focus. The other thing I really admire about her is that she's continued to educate herself and make herself a better human being, again and again and again. She just never stops learning, never stops growing. And that's why her career has staying power—because she conquers all her fears. If she hasn't done something, she tries it. She's not afraid of any challenge.

MADONNA ON JAMIE: No one knows more about music and movement than Jamie King. Working with him always pushes me to the limits of creativity. He is a true renaissance man with a beautiful heart.

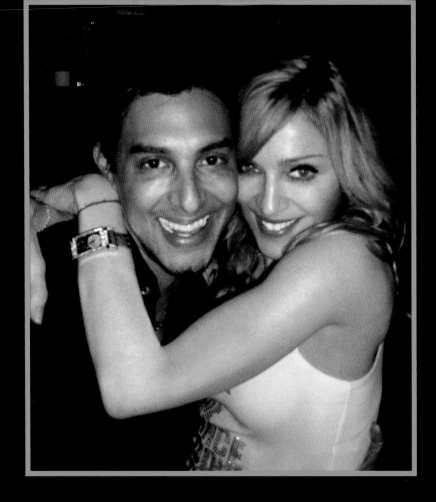

Jamie King and Madonna, supporters of Spirituality for Kids

Spirituality for Kids

I believe everything worthwhile starts with raising healthy and happy children. If they are taken care of physically and spiritually today, they will create a far better world tomorrow. That's why I contribute to the non-profit global organization Spirituality for Kids (SFK). Its goal is to end the suffering and chaos in children's lives around the world by giving them the tools of spirituality, tools that help them transform belief systems that limit their ability to realize their full potential and thus change their destiny.

I believe dance is spiritual, which is why I choose to share with the children of SFK the beauty of self-expression through movement. I know when I was young and having problems, dance was my outlet. I want these kids to also have dance as an option for an outlet.

Of course, dance isn't the only thing these children need. That's why I'm committed to donating a portion of the proceeds from this book to SFK. I encourage you to learn more about this amazing organization and make your own contribution by visiting its Web site at www.spiritualityforkids.org.

Remember, we all live in this world, so let's work together and make it a world we can be proud of.

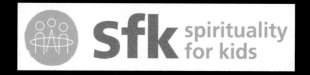

Part I

Rock Your Mind, Body, and Soul'

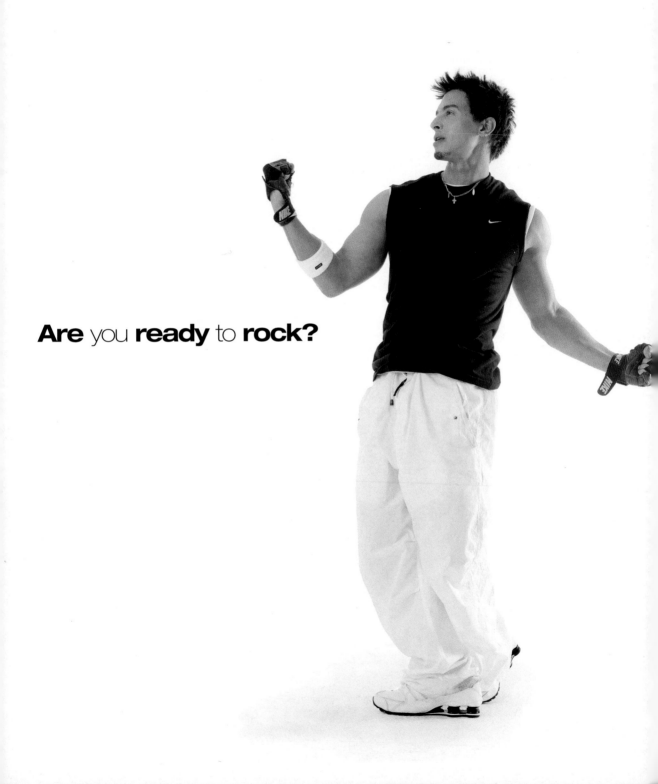

Are you **ready** to **rock?**

Chapter 1
Why Rock Your Body?

The easiest question anyone has ever asked me was: Why did you start dancing? The answer flew out before I could even process the question in my brain: Because I didn't have a choice. I was always dancing, maybe from the time I could walk. I can't remember a point in my life where I could say, okay, *here* is where I began dancing. Whenever I heard music, I danced. That's just who I was and who I still am.

Actually, if you ask any dancer this question, you'll likely get the same answer. Asking dancers why they dance is like asking a priest why he prays, or a mother why she loves her child. We do it because that's simply who we are. We do it to live. It's very simple, really, when you come right down to it—without dance, we would simply fade away to nothing.

I can hear you now . . . *But I'm not a dancer! I just want to get into better shape!*

I've got news for you—you *are* a dancer. All of us are. Without motion, without movement, we are nothing. The only difference between random movement and dance is where the movement comes from. With dance, the movement comes from within you—expressing a desire, telling a story, sending a message.

Because dancing is not just about dance steps. It's about your spirit, what you give, how you execute it through your soul. "Dancing is one of the best self-expressions that involves art," says Britney Spears. She should know—she's one of the top rock stars in the world. Dancing, she says, brings her "clarity, strength, and power."

I've worked with Britney from her very beginnings to her huge success as "Britney the

Pop Princess." During that time I've seen her mature as an artist and improve at her craft. That girl knows how to dance! Britney probably could have done just fine focusing on the voice end of things, but she's a lady who understands just how important dance is to pushing her career forward. She *gets* the power of dance and what it can do to propel a great performer into a huge star. She understands its power to turn her already exceptional music into a force that propels her audience to move and dance. Most important, she understands the spirit of dance.

Bottom line: Britney understands that dance is *everything*. It's storytelling, emotion, activity, cardio, strength training, endurance building. It's a sport and an art. A way to communicate without words. A therapy. A gathering. Dance is boogie and ballet, hip-hop and the hustle, rock 'n' roll and the rumba.

We dance for joy, dance in our seats, dance into a room. We boogie down, strut and spin, hip-hop and waltz. We watch dancers onstage and sit mesmerized before dancing flames. Without dance, we wouldn't have proms and cotillions, bands and ballrooms. Who knows what a stiller, smaller world we'd have without dance?

"Dance is a universal language," says my agent Julie McDonald. Julie began dancing when she was 5 years old. In the mid-1980s she founded the first agency to represent only dancers and choreographers. She created a whole new industry, and today, she and her partner, Tony Selznick, have competition from four or five such companies. During the years, she's seen dance come into its own, with the rebirth of the musical movie (*Chicago, Dreamgirls,* and *Stomp the Yard*), the dance shows on television (*So You Think You Can Dance* and *Dancing with the Stars*), and the explosion of live-performance extravaganzas both on the road and in venues like Las Vegas.

She thinks the appeal of dance comes from the fact that dance is a universal lan-

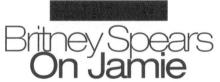

Britney Spears On Jamie

I love to work with Jamie King as a director and choreographer because he gets the big picture. Not many people do. Jamie is delightful to be around. He's sweet and sexy and there is always a mystery. Most important, he's not only brought me to the next level as an artist, but he also taught me to be fearless.

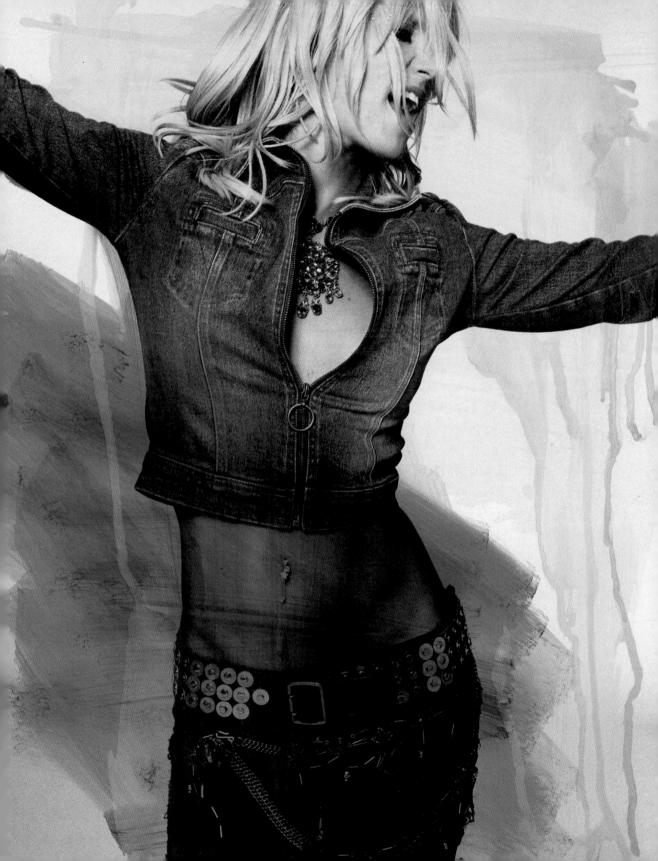

guage. "It speaks to people more than music," Julie says. "You don't need words, you don't need language of any kind—the body creates its own language, and when it's done right, it reaches people across all ages, class structures, and races. Dance just transcends every kind of barrier."

Okay, okay, I can hear you thinking . . . *Enough. What does this have to do with getting me in better shape and helping me lose weight?*

Everything. I don't want you to view Rock Your Body as *just* a fitness workout. It *is* that, but Rock Your Body is so much more. It's an introduction and an invitation into my world, a wonderful world, one I'm so lucky to be able to live in. It's a way to change every aspect of your life—not just your body—to find new ways to challenge your body and your limits. It's a journey—and I promise to hold your hand every step of the way.

This might seem a bit over the top for a fitness book, but bear with me here.

I've spent the past *15* years working with some of the top stars in the world—Michael Jackson, Prince, Madonna, Rain, Christina Aguilera, Ricky Martin, Pink, Shakira, Mariah Carey . . . even Ellen DeGeneres! I work 18-hour days, often 7 days a week. I've created the Nike Rockstar Workout, now taught in health clubs around the world, directed the top-grossing tour by a female artist in history (Madonna's 2006 *Confessions* tour, seen *in person* by 1.2 million people), and that kiss between Britney Spears, Madonna, and Christina Aguilera at the 2003 MTV Video Music Awards? Yup, that was me.

Why do I do this? Believe it or not, it's not for the money. It's for that unbelievable feeling I get when I express myself creatively. It's a high much higher than any drug could ever provide. It makes me feel sexy, confident, strong. The ability to have this feeling is a gift, I know, but it's a gift I now want to share with you. The gift of dance.

Read on to learn why you should use time and energy learning to Rock Your Body.

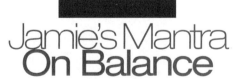

Jamie's Mantra
On Balance

Anything in life is about balance. I don't believe in overexercising, overeating, overdoing anything. Probably the only place in my life where I'm out of balance is work. I take on too much work—but I love it!

Rock Your Body for Eternal Youth

I think dance is the ultimate fountain of youth. I mean, look at Madonna. She looks and moves better than most 30-year-olds. She celebrated her 47th birthday by horseback riding (okay, she did fall and break her collarbone, hand, and ribs, but hey—at least she was *out there*!). Just a couple of months later she was shooting a music video even though her bones were still healing. You don't do that unless you're in amazing shape. And in the summer of 2006, of course, she broke all records with her *Confessions* world tour (which I directed), which was so successful she had to add dates to keep up with the demand.

Need more examples? How about Bette Midler, who turned 61 in December 2006 and, in my mind, remains the ultimate showgirl? How about Cher, who's 60, or Tina Turner, who is almost 70!

These women can move, dance, twirl, and compete with the best of anyone, regardless of age. Why? Because they're dancers. I really believe that the sheer physicality of the training they've had all these years has given them greater endurance and better health than "normal" people. They really are the ultimate divas.

But you don't have to be Madonna to reap the benefits of dance. Anyone who's a dancer—ballet, hip-hop, male, female—has an inner glow about them that shines through because they've found a way to express themselves. There is just no doubt about it: Dance is good for your mind, body, and soul.

(continued)

Rockin' at the Highest Levels

What does it take to get up there and dance as part of Madonna's backup, or as part of a music video, or behind Celine Dion in Las Vegas? Versatility, says fellow choreographer and friend Jeri Slaughter. I agree with him when he says, "To make it in this industry, you have to be a versatile dancer, able to adapt to any form of dance, whether it's jazz-based or hip-hop or break dancing or a combination of all three." So, for instance, you might find yourself break-dancing in a piece that also calls for a ballet pirouette. "But you don't have to be classically trained these days to make it," he says. And he's right. We've both worked with people whose only training occurred on the streets—and who did great.

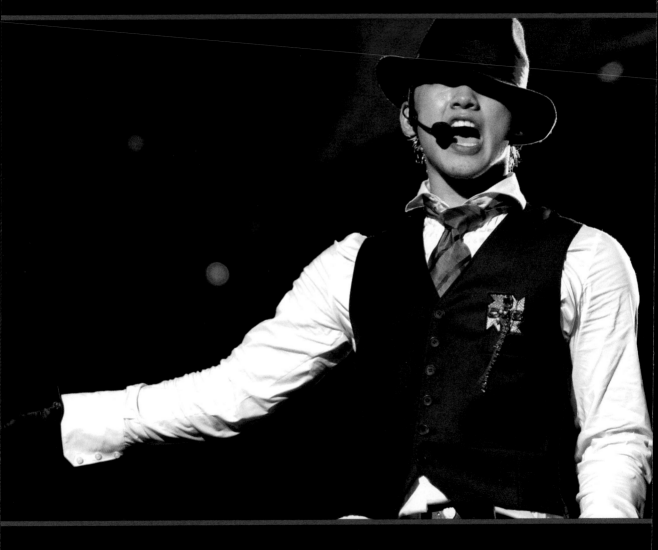

Rain

JAMIE ON RAIN: I've been working with Rain since 2006 and recently directed his *Rain's Coming* tour. It's no surprise to me that he's the number one music star throughout Asia, the most popular music star ever over there; no surprise that *Time* magazine voted him "the second most influential artist of 2006." Rain reminds me of Usher and Justin Timberlake with a little bit of Michael Jackson sprinkled in. He hits hard, with a mix of popping and strength and athleticism all rolled up into his hip-hop style. I view him as another representation of how dancers influence the world. He's a singer, but he uses dance to enhance his showmanship, to sell his music. He is just a clear example of how dance works to excite people and make them enthusiastic about a product.

RAIN ON JAMIE: Jamie is "one" with dance. His passion and love for dance is the reason I respect him so much. His experiences starting at a young age working with Prince to where he is today, working with the most famous artists in the world, have made him into a trendsetting director/choreographer. It is obvious that he invests a lot of effort into his work, but without his natural talent and unbelievable capabilities, all of his great achievements would have been impossible.

In fact, the benefits of dance on dancers are so strong that some dancers actually experience "withdrawal" symptoms like headaches, nervousness, and depression if they're forced to stop for injuries or other reasons.

Don't believe me? Listen to Britney: "Dancing gives you a sexy body as opposed to a boxy body from working out," she says. "It elongates you." And look at dancers, whether professional dancers on the stage or the amateurs you see on shows like *Dancing with the Stars*. Of course they have great bodies; they spend hours a day building long, lean muscle. But there's more to it than that. Dancers also stand taller, walk taller, move with a confidence often missing in most people. I guarantee you—stick with Rock Your Body and you'll have that confidence, too.

Another beauty is that you'll not only feel energized and fit after finishing the Rock Your Body workout, but you'll also feel sexy. I'm not kidding; I hear this from my dancers all the time. When they leave a Jamie King rehearsal, they feel sexy.

An added bonus—you'll get more hip. And no matter what your age, hipness is equated with youth. And with the growing dance craze as seen in movies like *Rize* and *You Got Served*, and the success of television shows like *Dancing with the Stars*, *The Ellen DeGeneres Show*, and *So You Think You Can Dance*, not to mention the huge popularity of MTV and VH1, there couldn't be a better time to start learning the coolest new moves.

These programs clearly show that America wants to get up and dance. They're proof that dance is inspirational, motivational, and highly addictive. What I love most

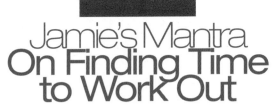

Jamie's Mantra
On Finding Time
to Work Out

I always make it part of my schedule to find time to rock my body so I can get the blood flowing and pumping and my heart going and stay in shape. If I don't get my daily workout in, I just don't feel right mentally. I need that hour to work out, to step away from everything else and get my body active. But it takes organization to find the time to work out. You have to schedule it in. You can't just hope it's going to happen, or put it at the bottom of the list and "try to fit it in."

about these types of shows is that they afford everybody—young and old—experienced or novice—male or female—the opportunity to show off their personal moves and style.

Rock It Out for Fitness

If you think dance doesn't make the cut as a sport, think again. As early as 1927, dance was recommended as "the most effective of all forms of exercise." In 1975, a study of 61 sports placed professional ballet second to football and just ahead of professional hockey in terms of its demand on the body and its need for speed, strength, and agility.

Today, many Olympic athletes use dance as part of their training to improve their control, agility, balance, and speed. And how about this: The International Olympic Committee granted "dancesport," a form of competitive ballroom dancing, as a provisional Olympic sport in 1997—the first step toward inclusion in the games themselves.

I first realized dance was a sport when I saw Gene Kelly dance. He was such a visionary, such an athletic dancer. Every time I've watched him dance in anything—a show, a movie, any presentation he's ever done—I've been amazed at the sheer athleticism he brings to dance, the way he was able to mix masculinity and dance, art and athleticism. His influence is part of what's shaped me into the kind of dancer, choreographer, and director I am today.

Another beautiful thing about dance is that unlike many workouts, you use your entire body—not just one muscle over and over again until it becomes fatigued. You're also not moving in just one direction over and over again, whether up and down or right to left. Instead, you're crossing over your body, turning around, twisting. You're using your body as it was meant to be used instead of in some artificial manner dreamed up by a fitness coach. Dance is the ultimate cross-training exercise.

One of the top producers/directors/choreographers in the field, Kenny Ortega (director and choreographer of the recent hit Disney Channel movie *High School Musical*), took tap dancing when he was a young boy and, more than 30 years later, says he still uses what he learned. "Dance puts you in a place of balance and grace in your life even if you don't dance professionally," he says. "It affects how I turn a corner, how I jump out of the way of something, my quick response to things."

(continued)

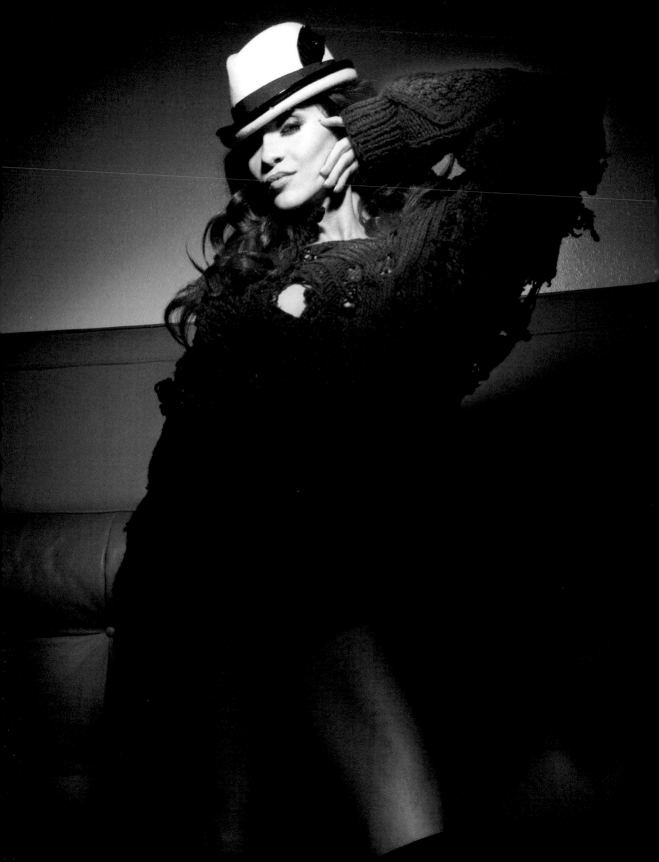

Pussycat Dolls'
Carmit Bachar

JAMIE ON CARMIT: *Carmit Bachar is one of the most visible dancers in the industry today, a member of the super-famous Pussycat Dolls. Born into a family of entertainers, she easily entered show business and has worked with some of the most successful artists in music, including No Doubt, Beyonce, P Diddy, Macy Gray, and Janet Jackson. She has numerous feature film credits, including* 13 Going on 30, Along Came Polly, The Scorpion King, *and* Charlie's Angels: Full Throttle. *Among her most recognized appearances was as Ricky Martin's "La Vida Loca" girl. Here are her thoughts on dance:*

"I've found through my worldwide touring with the Pussycat Dolls that dance is a universal language. You can always relate to people through dance. I was born with a cleft palate and cleft lip, so I had to learn very early to lose my self-consciousness. I was helped enormously by my parents. They showered me with love. But people would often say very brutal things, like 'What's wrong with your face?' When I told my agent about my dreams, he said, 'Don't get your hopes up and be prepared for a lot of rejection.' But I thought to myself, you know what? Screw that. I have a passion. I love what I'm doing and I'll continue to do it."

Julie Daugherty, physical therapist for the American Ballet Theater who works with some of the world's top dancers, can't say enough about the physical benefits of dance. "It's a great way to work on your fitness, and it can be a lot more fun than gym workouts," she says. "It also develops coordination, balance, and body awareness and can help you correct your posture." Plus, she says, it helps you with flexibility more than many other types of exercise while providing a great sense of accomplishment, which can boost your self-esteem.

Here is Julie's advice for new *and* old dancers:

- Begin any exercise routine slowly and carefully, and start at your own skill level. Don't force anything. Work on your flexibility first, in order to safely develop your range of motion, and then build your strength within that range of motion.
- Always warm up and take time to stretch afterward.
- Drink enough fluid.
- Don't do too much too soon. That's when you strain a muscle or get an overuse injury like tendonitis. And if you're tired and haven't warmed up sufficiently, that's when you're most likely to hurt yourself.
- Find a balance between cardio workouts, strengthening, flexibility, and something that helps to reduce stress. Many dancers find a daily ballet class can be a form of meditation—it is very structured and requires intense focus on steps and their bodies.

"No matter what kind of dance you do," Julie says, "you'll learn about and appreciate the art and vocabulary of dance, and often the accompanying music as well. Dance is not just a physical activity—it has an important cultural aspect as well. It broadens your view and appreciation of the world."

My agent Tony Selznick calls dance more "inspiring" than any other exercise. "It compels you to get better," he says. "Yoga is great and personal, but there's something about dance that just excites you and makes you feel part of a bigger picture."

"Dance is very important in my life and in keeping me fit because I don't have time to go to the gym and work out," says pop singer Rihanna, who, not coincidentally, was named Billboard Music Awards Female Artist of the Year in 2006. "Sometimes it's the only exercise I get."

"It's amazing how quickly I slim down on tour because of the dancing," says R&B

Jamie's Mantra
On Developing the Mind-Set of an Athlete

To me, the mind-set of an athlete is composed of four things: will, strength, conviction, and commitment. *Will* means that once you set your mind to doing something, you can do anything. *Strength* refers not only to physical strength but also to the mental strength to carry on beyond where your physical strength gets you. And everything depends on your having the *conviction* to follow through on your dreams and the *commitment* to stick with your quest even when you think you can't go another step, especially when you're confronted with failure. You also have to believe in yourself, believe that you're a winner. And compete with yourself. If you did a 30-minute high-endurance workout today, do 35 minutes tomorrow. Or do it better. Or do it differently. But never settle for just good enough.

singer-songwriter Pink, with whom I've also worked. "It's incredible exercise and really fun, too. Better than the boring gym!"

Television personality and supermodel Tyra Banks says she actually dances on the treadmill in the gym. "I'll be rockin' out to Beyonce's 'Deja-Vu' or Fergie's 'Fergalicious' and channeling the whole video in my mind . . . and thinking I'm re-creating it during my run. I mean, I look crazy . . . but it makes 60 minutes feel like 10!"

She even has "dance offs" with her makeup artist and her stylist. "We make up routines and get all sexy out on the dance floor . . . or right there in my dressing room."

And as my friend and fellow choreographer Mia Michaels says, "I'm 6 feet tall and a woman of some size, but my muscle tone is so firm because of dancing. When I dance, I feel like I weigh 2 pounds."

Another friend, Mari Winsor, who created Winsor Pilates, says she loves dance as an exercise option because it "flows." "There are many benefits to constant motion without stopping," she says. "Your heart rate will increase, allowing you to burn calories and lose weight, and you will be more flexible, stronger, more coordinated, and more graceful."

"Dance has always been like sport, and it only gets more athletic over time," says my mentor Joe Tremaine, who has worked with just about every major star in the

(continued)

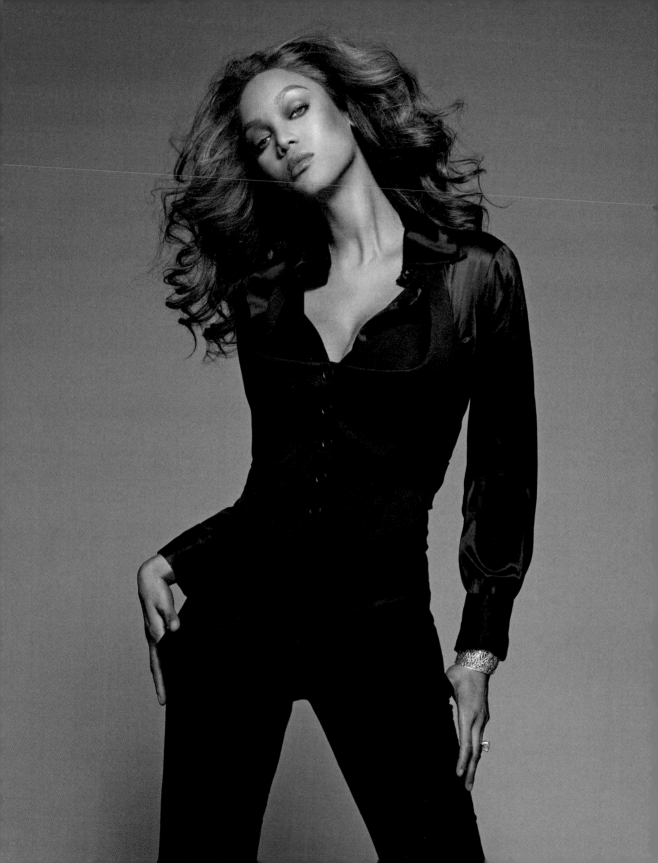

Tyra Banks

JAMIE ON TYRA: Supermodel Tyra Banks of the *Tyra Banks Show* says she knew from the first moment she met me that we had to work together. I felt the same way. She is an incredibly inspirational woman, a real superstar. What I learned from working with her is that she loves dance. Most people don't think of models as dancers, but they are because they commit movement to music, especially on a runway in front of a crowd. Nobody works the runway like Tyra.

TYRA ON JAMIE: I had an idea for a live show and had just seen Jamie's work on Madonna's latest masterpiece—her *Confessions* tour. There is nothing I appreciate more than someone who can take a creative vision—a seed of an idea—and bring it to life fluidly and brilliantly. Jamie does just this as a director. Adding layers of color, smoke, art, music, sexuality, and depth—Jamie makes things *pop* off a page and aligns music with visuals—crafting it all into a story. He blew me away. I mean, his instincts are just incredible!

business. "Look at basketball and football and tennis and all the others. It's all about body awareness and making the best use of your movements. The smartest athletes always get themselves in dance classes."

You can also burn about 400 calories during a 1-hour hip-hop class or workout like Rock Your Body. Do the workout three times a week and that's a whopping 1,200 calories. If you keep everything else the same, i.e., you don't suddenly turn into a cheesecake addict, by the end of the year you could lose 17 pounds—while having fun!

Just remember: Dance is much more than a workout. That's why I want you to embrace the world of dance throughout the day, not just when you're doing the Rock Your Body performance. I want you to dance everywhere. In the shower (careful, don't slip!), in your bedroom, waiting at a cross walk. I want you to start taking what you learn through my workout, along with your new body, to clubs. Instead of sitting at the table like a boring dud during weddings, I want you to get out there on the floor and dance. Move your body!

Rock Your Body for Health

I know you bought this book in part because you want to lose weight. And you *will* lose weight. Heck, you can even lose weight ballroom dancing, as you might have seen on *Dancing with the Stars*. Pro football player and *Dance* winner Emmitt Smith dropped 16 pounds while on the show.

But forget about the weight for a minute; think about your overall health. For instance,

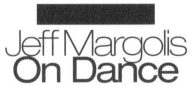

Jeff Margolis On Dance

Award-winning producer-director Jeff Margolis has shaped more than 100 of the entertainment industry's biggest events, including the Academy Awards. His production company produced the NBC dramatic series Fame, which had such a great impact on me. "As a director of entertainment television, the art of dance gives me the ability to capture movement and paint visual images for the audience," Jeff says. "I find that working with dancers is one of the most stimulating and fulfilling opportunities offered today."

when 35 people in Rhode Island danced for exercise, their overall heart rate, physical fitness, and muscle tone improved just as much as those who followed a walking/jogging program. Another study of 110 heart patients found waltzing worked just as well at improving their endurance as cycling or walking on the treadmill.

Here's a secret: Even though the researchers didn't say so, I can guarantee the dancers had more fun than the cyclers or walkers.

Why? Because dance is so much fun! "It's light, it lifts you up, it gives you a high," says my agent Julie McDonald. "I know so many people who started dancing as a hobby, and they end up becoming addicted to it."

It's more than "just" exercise. "It's dancing for fun, for health—to change your world," she says.

And, in fact, dance is often used to change peoples' worlds, helping them improve their body image and handle mental health issues like depression and anxiety.

It's called dance therapy, and while hospitals, nursing homes, and other medical facilities use it for ill patients, I believe it's something you can incorporate into a healthy lifestyle.

Think about it. Man has been using dance as a healing therapy since the first human (or humanlike being) walked on two legs. Just consider the rich history of dance within cultures much older than ours—Asian yoga, qigong, and tai chi therapies are all dance-based, their beginnings dating back to Taoist monks who learned ways to breathe and move designed to promote mental clarity and physical strength. In fact, dance is frequently mentioned in old medical writings as a way to release hidden and "pent-up" emotions.

The field of "dance therapy" itself grew from dancers' own efforts to prevent or heal injuries and, later, to work through various physical and mental problems in the best way they knew how. Even though the official name is "dance therapy," I prefer to call it "movement therapy," and I urge you to go beyond the routines in Rock Your Body to find the movements that work best for you.

How?

Mari Winsor

JAMIE ON MARI: When it comes to health and fitness, Mari Winsor is an athletic guru. She invented Winsor Pilates, a unique and hugely successful workout program. I'm so flattered that she's participating in my quest to get the world dancing, because she truly knows how to sculpt a body.

MARI ON JAMIE: Jamie King is one of the most exciting and innovative directors and choreographers of our generation. He has choreographed some of the best-looking stars in show business. His Rock Your Body workout is sure to bring out the best in you!

Start by becoming aware of your body. Stand in a quiet room, holding yourself straight, shoulders back, chin lifted. Close your eyes and listen to your body. What part of your body do you hear? Is it your back, crying out with pain from yesterday's 2-hour drive? Your neck, aching from the 8 hours you spent hunched over a keyboard? Your psyche, sad over some pain you can't seem to remember?

How would that feeling express itself as a movement? If it's your back, for instance, perhaps you want to bend over from the waist, your arms hanging down, and swing side-to-side like an elephant swings its trunk. Don't be afraid and don't be embarrassed. After all, there is no one to see you. This is between you and your body.

As you move, pay attention to your breathing and to the individual parts of your body. What are you feeling? What does the movement make you think about? By focusing on your breathing as you move, you are performing a form of meditation, moving your mind/body closer together, which, as we know, is a form of healing in and of itself. In fact, the very premise of dance therapy is related to the idea that the mind and body work in conjunction with one another.

That's one reason dance therapy is used so often with cancer patients and those with chronic pain: because dance gives you a sense of control. And loss of control is a major component in the stress associated with illness as well as pain. It's a well-known fact that pain is worse when you feel you have no control over it. That's why natural childbirth educators train women to focus on their breathing—it gives them control over some aspect of their bodies so the pain doesn't sweep them helplessly along.

Dance provides that same feeling of control through its sense of the spiritual and its mastery of movement.

With this feeling of control, your own sense of helplessness and fear abate somewhat. As they fade, so does the pain.

Celebrities I've Worked With: Michael Jackson

I consider Michael Jackson one of my earliest teachers. As the youngest dancer on his *Dangerous* world tour in the 1990s (actually, his backup dancer), I was a sponge. I was so lucky to be able to learn from the ultimate showman—the King of Pop himself. I learned how to perform on a grand scale, how to make spectacle, how to be the ultimate showman. One other thing I learned from him: Never let down your audience and always give 100 percent.

Using Dance to Heal

Just how is dance being used as part of the healing arts? How about . . .

- To strengthen the immune system through moderate exercise.

- To reduce the pain associated with conditions like chronic fatigue syndrome and fibromyalgia.

- As part of a holistic treatment for eating disorders.

- To reduce test anxiety. In one study of 29 young men, those participating in four 35-minute movement sessions over 2 weeks showed lower levels of self-reported test anxiety than a control group that didn't undergo the movement therapy.

- To improve the quality of life for breast cancer patients, as well as improve their body image.

Other health benefits of Rock Your Body:

- **Boost your cardiovascular fitness.** Everyday tasks, such as carrying your backpack, lugging groceries, or running up the stairs, will suddenly feel easier because your heart will be stronger and your lung capacity will have increased. You'll have more energy and be quicker and more agile. And when you get on the dance floor, you'll find that many of the moves you've been following to get in shape have given you the ability and confidence to move like a rock star!

- **Build strength and define your muscles.** Dancing is a total-body workout. After a few weeks of the Rock Your Body workout, you'll see your abs tighten and the muscles in your legs and arms become more defined. Every part of your body will become firmer.

- **Improve your overall health.** The aerobic and strength-training elements of dance have been shown to help lower cholesterol and blood pressure, reduce the risk of diabetes and heart disease, and improve fatigue. You'll build stronger bone because dance is a weight-bearing activity. And, because you'll feel better about your body, you'll probably find your sex life gets, well, sexier!

- **Change your body composition.** Because my workout is an endurance workout—aerobic movement for 20 minutes or more—your body will burn fat during the routines. Within 6 to 8 weeks of doing the workout 3 or 4 hours a week, you should see your percentage of body fat decline.

Laurie Ann Gibson

JAMIE ON LAURIE ANN:

I first met choreographer Laurie Ann Gibson when I was choreographing a routine for Salt-N-Pepa for the Grammys and she was one of the dancers. Since then, she's choreographed the motion picture *Honey* as well as MTV's *Making the Band,* danced on *In Living Color,* and developed routines for stars including Hilary Duff. Here's what Laurie Ann recalls about the first time we worked together.

LAURIE ANN ON JAMIE:

Jamie had this four count of eight, but the time in which he wanted us to do it was impossible. I said, "How do you expect me to get down and up in that amount of time?" Jamie, true to form, didn't get angry or sarcastic. He just gently told me, "Honey, I know you can do it."

Jamie is every choreographer's choreographer. He has this gift inside him to transform you. It's as if he's saying to you, "The world may tell you that you can't, but I'm going to encourage you to do what you never thought you could do." And when he does that, he literally defies gravity.

If you stop to think about what he's teaching you, you'll never believe you can get there, but he teaches you in such a way that you don't even realize you're committing to the movements that he's creating until you walk out of the rehearsal and you're like, "I can't believe I just did that!" and you feel championed by the fact that you were able to do it."

Rock It for Self-Expression

As you probably already figured out from my rant in the beginning of this chapter, dance is much more than just a good workout. It's the same for most of the stars I work with, like Rihanna. "For me, dance is an expression," she says. "It's part of the importance of music in my life." Tell me more, I say.

"I've always loved music, and when I hear music, I automatically want to dance," she explains. Part of this is her upbringing, she says. "In Barbados if you can't dance, it's a disgrace. It comes very naturally and is very cultural." So she was raised learning to express her emotions through dance.

And here's where she says something else I firmly believe: "Dance doesn't have to be choreographed," she says. "It's just movement, and you should have a good time while doing it."

Even with Rock Your Body?

Yes, she says. "You don't have to learn to do it to a certain count or a certain way; it's simply movement that you enjoy doing to music."

That's also how fellow choreographer Laurie Ann Gibson describes dance. "For me, dance is the freedom to be who you are internally in your spirit and your soul," she says. "It's a language that, once you give into it, helps you become more confident."

More confident?

"Sure. Because dancers don't speak with their voices, they speak with their bodies." So learning to dance, whether professionally or for fun or fitness, "teaches you to be bold, to be fearless, to walk into a room and be okay with how your body enters the room, how you sit down, what that body language is . . . Dance is a really powerful means of communication."

"Dance is an expression," says friend and choreographer Jeri Slaughter. "It lets you release whatever mood you're in with the outer movement of your body, your outer spirit." The beauty of dance as a way to get fit, says Jeri, is that "it's something you can have fun doing and not have to worry about doing it correctly. You can just be free and open and express what you're feeling and express your spirit and just go for it rather than having to specifically lift a weight and try to run on the treadmill."

Plus, he says, dance is both more therapeutic and more spiritual than any other kind of physical activity. "You can feel free, have fun, smile, laugh, and learn, all at once."

Jeri Slaughter

JAMIE ON JERI: I first met Jeri Slaughter when he auditioned for me as a young dancer. Since then, he's choreographed music videos for a variety of stars, including Christina Aguilera, Kelly Osbourne, and Shania Twain. **JERI ON JAMIE:** The thing that most impresses me about Jamie is how quickly he moves. He can do that because he knows what he wants. He has a vision already in his head, and basically he wants everyone to get that vision and get it fast. That's helped a lot of dancers or anyone he works with to move forward to get things done and move on rather than procrastinate. Some other choreographers come in not knowing what they're doing, without any vision. Jamie's vision is what sets him apart.

"Dance has always helped me deal with life," says Carmen Electra, one of Hollywood's most versatile personalities. Carmen, who has starred in numerous films, including *Cheaper by the Dozen 2, Starsky and Hutch,* and *Nothing but the Truth,* has her own dance troupe and released her own DVD workout series, *Aerobic Striptease.* I first met her when we worked together with Prince in the early '90s, and I've worked on several projects with her since.

"I've been dancing since I was 5," she says. "I was a shy kid, and what I loved about dance was that I didn't have to use words. I still feel the same way to some extent. Dance has been my outlet, a release when I go through painful experiences."

And Pink, the R&B singer-songwriter-turned-actress whom I've directed, says this about dance: "When you can close your eyes and let your body go, there's no better feeling in the world."

(continued)

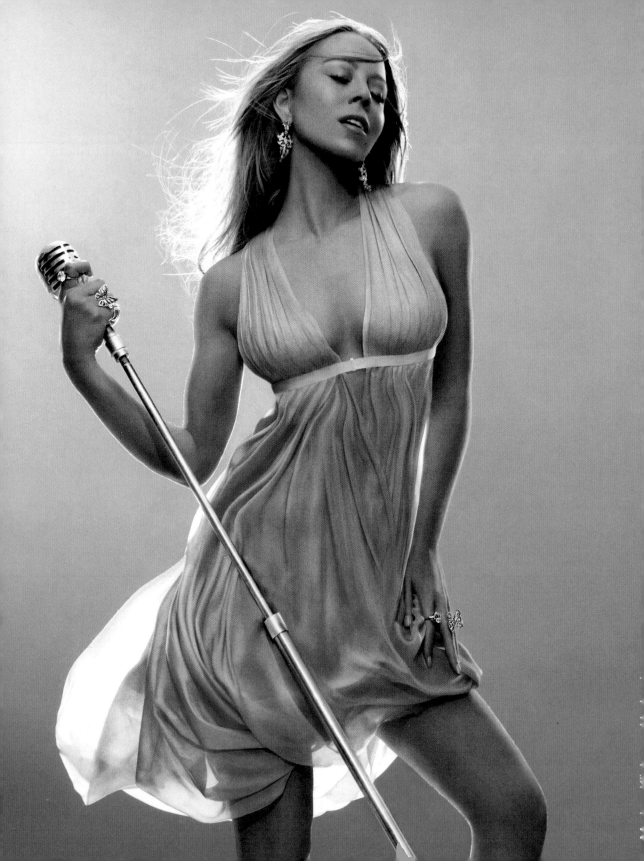

Mariah Carey

JAMIE ON MARIAH: Mariah Carey is a legend, pure and simple. She's got the gift of voice and song, and she's an amazing songwriter. She's also a survivor, a comeback kid, which is something I really love. She's gone up, then she's come down, then she's gone way, way up. And she keeps going. I just so admire that in people if they can go through a negative time and come out on top. She oozes sensuality . . . and those legs!

MARIAH ON JAMIE: Working with Jamie King is always a pleasure. His talent as a director/choreographer is obvious, but his real gift is in creating a comfortable environment for artists to work in. He has an innate ability to give my songs movement. He is not only fabulous himself, but he assists others in becoming an even more fabulous version of themselves.

Rockin' for a New Life

If someone tells me they don't like the way they look, I have one question for them: "Why?"

Why don't you like the way you look, and what are you going to do about it? Often the person starts babbling about a big butt and thunder thighs and an overhanging belly. That's when I say hold on. When was the last time you looked, really *looked,* at your body? No, I'm not talking about the disgusted glance you gave it while trying on bathing suits in a poorly lighted dressing room. I'm talking about stripping naked and standing in front of a full-length mirror. Come on, you can do it.

Now open your eyes. What do you see? Don't focus on the flaws; instead, seek out the strengths. Notice that long line from your neck to your shoulders that continues down your arms. See the gracefulness of your arms as you raise and lower them. Even if they're not tightly toned, I bet you can still see the muscles in your upper arms and shoulders.

Now look at your hips and waist. Honor them for what they are. Twist yourself halfway around and back, bend over and touch the floor with your hands (if you can; if not, just bend as far as you can). Watch how your body obeys your commands, how it was built to move.

Now move down to your legs. Lift each leg straight up, then lift each leg up with a bended knee. Feel the hidden strength within your legs? Say a silent "thank you" for having such strong legs that can get you through your hectic day, even if the only walking you do is up and down the stairs and to and from the parking lot. These are the legs that are going to rock for you.

Now look at your feet. I'll admit, feet are not the most beautiful things (especially dancers' feet). But think about the pounding they take every day, and you can understand why calluses and bunions are not something to be despised but something to be applauded. They're signs of the work those feet do nearly every minute of every day.

The point of this exercise is to get you to stop looking at your body as a thing that needs to be fixed or changed, and instead view it as an instrument totally within your power and ability to play. Through the routines in Rock Your Body, you'll learn how to tune that instrument and play more advanced pieces than you ever thought possible.

Once you begin dancing, I promise you'll find that the way you hold yourself, the way you walk, sit, stand, even the way your clothes fit, will change—whether or not you lose any weight.

These changes will all come from a heightened awareness of your body and where it exists in space. Instead of viewing your body as some schlumpy thing you have to haul around, you'll begin to feel one with your body. For the first time in your life, I bet you find yourself actually *fitting* into your body instead of feeling that it's some alien thing you've been burdened with.

You'll find yourself standing taller, your spine straighter, holding your stomach in without being aware of it. You'll find your chin tilted up just that tiny bit extra to make your neck look 5 inches longer. You'll stop bumping into things because, as you become more aware of how your body fits into space, you'll become more graceful.

That's why I believe that dance is a way of living, not just a fitness activity. For instance, nowhere in this book will you find me telling you to use dance *just* to lose weight or *only* to stay in shape. Sure, I want you to use dance as a way to stay active. If you're active—no matter what your weight or shape—you'll be much healthier than if the only movement you get is shuffling from the couch to the kitchen. But the main reason I want you to dance is because it can literally change your life.

Unfortunately, we seem to have lost that reverence for dance, for movement. As Peter Martins, former ballet master in chief of the New York City Ballet, wrote: "We're a society that perpetuates stillness." He is so right. Most of us spend our days in front of computers or in other stationary jobs. Even though we've become more immersed than ever in music, thanks to the ubiquitous iPod and other MP3 players, when is the last time you saw someone actually swaying or

Benny Medina

JAMIE ON BENNY: Benny is a legendary producer and manager of superstar artists including Mariah Carey and Tyra Banks. **BENNY ON JAMIE:** I'm a manager, and Jamie King is my "go-to guy" for any artist I work with. Jamie has the ability to focus on the entire scope of a show, from the smallest of details to the grandest of concepts. His ability to work with an artist and, through his skill and passion, create the definitive representation of that artist to the audience is unparalleled. Jamie King is "the answer" to any show.

tapping or moving his body to the sound that must be pouring through the earbuds? We sit or stand with plugs in our ears, pouring music into ourselves but allowing it no path of exit.

Now, with Rock Your Body, that music will have a way to come out.

Rockin' Away the Stress

Here's another reason to dance—to help your body manage the myriad stresses that get thrown at it every day. Dance *helping* with stress? Right about now you're shaking your head, saying, "Jamie, dude, this dancing thing is stressing me out because I can't get the steps right."

Hey, don't worry about getting the steps "right." This is between you and you—no one is judging you, watching you, or expecting anything out of you other than that you try.

Now, back to the stress thing. You've probably heard before about the way your body responds to stress. Whenever you encounter a stressor, whether it's your boss yelling at you because your project is late, your kid's babysitter calling in sick 2 minutes before you leave for work, or your mother finding out she has breast cancer, your body reacts the same way. It's immediately flooded with stress hormones like cortisol and norepinephrine that send out chemical signals to various parts of your body so it can "flee" or "fight."

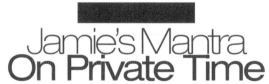

Jamie's Mantra
On Private Time

You know, I spend a lot of my time surrounded by people. Dancers, performers, managers, agents . . . and I bet you do too. How often do you get time alone? Well, I want you to do what I do—make yourself a priority for at least 30 minutes a day. It can be quiet time when you're sitting in a room reading or thinking, or it can be the time you do the Rock Your Body workout. Just know that this time is for you. It's for your mental stability, your way of taking your goals and desires and plan of attack and thinking about and focusing on them. But most important, it's a way to recharge your batteries. If you don't do this, I guarantee you will burn out.

As a result, your liver releases glucose, or sugar, to give your muscles energy; your circulatory system directs blood away from your gut toward your arms and legs so you can run or fight; your heart beats faster to pump more blood; your breathing rate quickens to bring in more oxygen; and—here's the kicker—your immune system sends out inflammatory cells to repair any damage you experience as you're fighting or fleeing.

This is all great if you're actually fighting or fleeing, but come on, how likely are you to get into it in the shopping center parking lot?

Instead, you're having this over-the-top reaction 10, 20, or more times a day simply as a reaction to the stresses in your life. Over time, as you might imagine, this wreaks havoc on every part of your body. All that extra glucose? It has nowhere to go, so it builds up in your bloodstream, which signals your pancreas to make more insulin to get that glucose into cells. Eventually, those overstuffed cells say "no more," and the glucose turns into fat, usually around your middle.

Those inflammatory chemicals? They're still hanging out in your bloodstream, only with no real damage to repair, they sit around doing their own damage to blood vessels and other tissues, increasing your risk of heart disease, depression, and other chronic conditions.

So how does dance help with all this?

Exercise—any kind of exercise—is a known antidote for stress. It provides an outlet for the pent-up energy that comes from tamping down

(continued)

Kenny Ortega

JAMIE ON KENNY:

Kenny Ortega is an Emmy award-winning producer, director, and choreographer. He's choreographed numerous movies, including *Dirty Dancing, Ferris Bueller's Day Off,* and *Pretty in Pink.* He also directed and choreographed the Disney Channel made-for-television movie *High School Musical,* one of the most successful original Disney Channel movies ever made. I first met Kenny when I auditioned for Michael Jackson's *Dangerous* tour, which he was directing. Like Debbie Allen, Kenny went from dancer to choreographer, to director of film and stage, and I greatly respect his obvious talent.

KENNY ON JAMIE: I still remember the first time I saw Jamie. My casting director, Greg Smith, pulled me aside and said, "Get ready. You're going to see someone who is going to knock your socks off." It is only once in every great while you find yourself in a room with someone where you immediately realize how special this person is. I felt it the first time Leonardo DiCaprio read for me on a film project. And I felt it when I met Jamie. He just lit up the whole space. He was alien to everything I'd ever seen. Just his look and his energy. And then when he danced . . . there was a kind of energy that shot out from him. He just cut through the space. I couldn't move fast enough to secure him for a role on the tour.

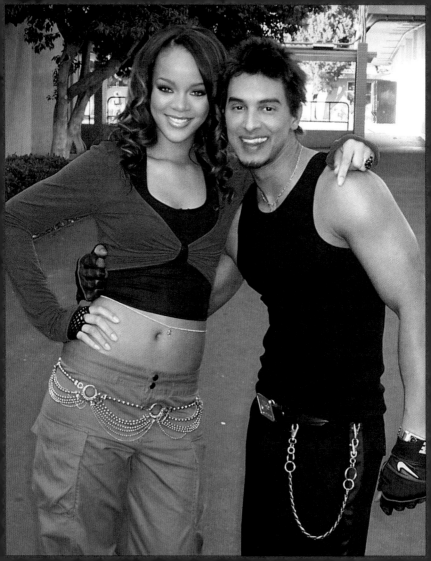

Rihanna

JAMIE ON RIHANNA: When I was hired to create and direct the Nike Rockstar Workout, I immediately thought of Rihanna, named America's Teen Choice Awards' Breakthrough Female Artist and R&B Artist of the Year in 2006. The Nike campaign was about dance fitness, and I wanted to select a young, exciting, athletic music star who could dance. At the time, Rihanna was just up-and-coming, but I knew she was going to be highly influential on the music scene. We chose her song "SOS" prior to its release as the soundtrack. She was a delight to work with. She was so inspired by my dance workout. She really understood what I was going for—the validation of dance as fitness. Together, we created an inspirational campaign to get viewers off their butts and into shape.

RIHANNA ON JAMIE: He pulled stuff out of me that I didn't know I had. I'd heard of him long before the commercial and was already a big fan of his work. Such a big fan, in fact, that when I learned he'd be the creative director of the Nike Rockstar Workout commercial, I found myself nervous about working with him. But I shouldn't have worried. It was very easy and fun and that's important. In fact, Jamie makes all his choreography fun, whether it's for a rock star like me or for someone looking to get in shape with the Rock Your Body routine.

One thing about Jamie: He never stops. Even on the set for the Nike Rockstar Workout, I would catch him lifting weights between rehearsal sets. Everyone else is sitting down, catching their breath, drinking water, and there's Jamie pumping iron. He is incredible.

Questions You Wanted to Ask about Rock Your Body but Were Afraid To

So here they are, asked and answered.

Q: Am I too old to dance hip-hop?

Absolutely not! Can you move? Do you like to listen to music with a strong beat?
Do you like having fun? Then you're never too old to dance hip-hop—or any
other type of dance, for that matter.

Q: Will I really lose weight dancing?

Holy cardio, Batman! Will you ever! And the more you give, the more you
put out, the better the result will be.

Q: Is it hard to remember the choreography?

Not at all, because you are supposed to go at your own pace. Learn the steps as slowly or as
quickly as you want. Add your own steps, or ignore my steps altogether and simply move to
the music for the hour. But really, once you learn the basics, the rest is just repetition.

Q: Do my moves have to be exact?

Not unless you're auditioning for the next Jennifer Lopez music video! These moves are for
you, no one else. Make them your own!

**Q: Do I have to do any other exercise if I'm doing the Rock Your Body workout three
times a week?**

That's really up to you. But if you're completing the entire workout three times a week, you're
getting a great overall workout, cardio *and* strength training, and you can consider your
exercise needs met!

Q: Do I have to follow the Dancer's Diet?

Hey, you don't have to do anything. But if you want to reap all the benefits of the Rock Your
Body workout, then yes, you have to follow the Dancer's Diet. It's designed to provide the
nutritional power you need to keep up with the workout along with the micro- and macronutrients you require to build strong muscle and bone without packing on the pounds.

your inner desire to fight or flee, adds muscle cells so there's more muscle to take up that excess blood sugar, and releases other hormones that turn off the inflammatory process. It allows you to express your emotions, instead of keeping them inside, and discharges energy throughout your body.

One reason dance helps so much when it comes to stress is that dance provides that sense of control we talked about earlier. After all, *you* are in control in terms of where you move your body, how you move your body, what you choose to express. Dance itself often requires tight control over your body, with your stomach held in, your head held high, only certain muscles allowed to move.

Compare that to the rest of your life where you probably feel as out of control as an 18-wheeler with no brakes careening down a mountain. Think about it—how much control do you have at work? At home? In your financial dealings, in terms of how your body looks, in terms of how you feel physically? This out-of-control stress is the worst kind of stress to have.

But dance . . . ahhh. That sense of control it returns to you gradually expands from the hour a day you're actually dancing to the rest of your life, beginning with how you look and feel.

Just ask my manager and producer Daniel Sladek, who over the years has represented the careers of acclaimed actors, directors, and dancers including Tony Award Best Actor nominee Adam Cooper, star of Matthew Bourne's hit West End /Broadway sensation *Swan Lake,* and Rasta Thomas, star of Broadway's Billy Joel/Twyla Tharp hit *Movin Out.* How does he deal with his stress managing my career? He hits the dance floor! "Before I realized who Jamie was professionally, I would see him out dancing and knew I somehow wanted to work with him," says Daniel. "His spirit on the dance floor is powerfully addictive. I believe if you dance powerfully, you work and live powerfully. Dance is a way of life."

But, Jamie, you're still saying, *I'm not a dancer.* Oh yes, you are. And in the next chapter, I'm going to tell you exactly why you are.

Celebrities I've Worked With: Prince

Prince was a huge influence in my life. I mean, I used to dress up like him when I was young! He was my teacher. He taught me how to match music and movement and make them one. He taught me about staging, lighting, and editing. Among the many things I love about him are his attention to detail and his perfectionism, not to mention how he's an innovator.

Keep **moving.**
Keep **grooving.**
Create your **own**
personal **style.**

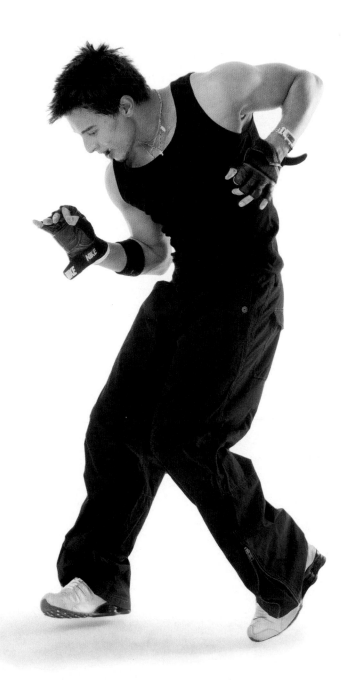

Chapter 2
Unleashing
Your Inner Rock Star

I'm curious. Why did you buy this book? Why didn't you pick up a workout book that focused on Pilates, or aerobics, or any of the dozens of other approaches out there? I think I know why. Because you know—and I know—that somewhere deep within you is a dancer. Now is your chance to bring him or her out into the open.

Nonetheless, I bet you're scared. Scared of messing up, scared you won't be able to do it, scared you've made a terrible—albeit not very expensive—mistake. Relax. Let me make one thing very clear: Everyone can dance. Say it after me: Everyone can dance. Say it again. And again. Only by getting you past your negativity, whether it's about your body, having the time to dance, or being able to move to the music, will you ever really be able to benefit from the Rock Your Body workout.

For I believe that inside every person is a dancer. Even if you're in a wheelchair, you can still dance. Because dance is freedom of expression; it's movement to music, whether that music is in your environment or inside your head. You can dance to the sound of wind. To the sound of a woodpecker in the woods. I mean, think about it: Dance is the oldest form of human expression on the planet. Dance is universal in every culture from the beginning of time. There's simply no such thing as a bad dancer. Dance is too personal, too spiritual. It belongs to the individual, and only the individual—that would be you—can judge its quality.

Nonetheless, my friend Mari Winsor, creator of Winsor Pilates, says she often hears, "Well, but *I'm not a dancer.*"

"I think Jamie and I agree, everyone's a dancer," Mari says. "We all have our own special rhythm, and though you may not be able to mimic a trained dancer, some-where inside you your own spirit and personality can shine through and make you feel amazing."

You're never too old to dance, either. My grandmother, who lives in a retirement community in Arizona, is still dancing, participating in a soft-shoe tap troupe. It amazes me. But that's how she finds her enjoyment. It's a communal activity that helps her stay healthy and fit and continue to love life.

And don't tell me you feel embarrassed out there. What do you mean *embar-rassed*? I want you to "dance as if nobody's watching," as Sting wrote, but really, no one *is* watching!

But I also want you to ask yourself *why* you're embarrassed. Is it because you think your body is too big to dance? Because you're afraid you'll mess up the steps? Because you're not used to letting go and simply feeling instead of thinking all the time? All of these reasons—and any others you may have—are exactly the reason why you need the Rock Your Body workout! Committing to this program will enable you to get past your fears (and, after all, what is embarrassment but shame at our own fears?) and excel. It will enable you to turn your weaknesses into strengths.

Just listen to what my friend and fellow choreographer Mia Michaels has to say. Mia, who was nominated for an Emmy for her choreography of Celine Dion's *A New Day* show in Las Vegas, talks about dance as a "mind, body, and soul" activity. "I think dance is the most freeing, healthiest way to get in shape because it moves you to another place," she says. "Dance is a gift that God gave everybody, and it's up to us what we do with it. But I think part of our humanness is to dance. If everyone danced, I think there would be no war."

When she's dancing, she adds, "I'm a completely different person. I feel like the most beautiful, the most powerful, the most exquisite being on the earth because I get lost in the movement."

That's an important point: getting lost in the movement. What Mia means by this is that you can transcend the steps and the choreography and just feel the movement and the music. When you do that, she says, dance becomes "like a drug. It just takes you to a place you allow yourself to go."

Actress and dancer Carmen Electra says she used to think you needed technique to be a dancer. "Now I'd say it takes passion, heart, and soul," she says. "You don't need technique—although it's always good to have. But you do have to want to reach out and make people feel what you feel."

Dance is also empowering, says my friend and fellow choreographer Laurie Ann Gibson. "You empower yourself by understanding how and what type of language your body can speak," she says.

And she strongly believes that anyone can dance—even if they've never moved to the music before in their life. "There's a dancer in every single person," she says. "It's just about taking the first step." To find that hidden dancer, she, like my client Rihanna, urges you to stop worrying about the challenge of the steps or the dance itself. "Go with the feeling," Laurie Ann says. "How does that move make you feel?" Once you find the feeling, she says, "The feeling will become the steps."

(continued)

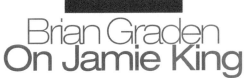

Brian Graden
On Jamie King

Jamie King is the first person I remember who said, "I'm not a director or choreographer as much as I'm an entertainment experience producer. You can't really separate the choreography from the set, from the environment, from the musicality . . . I imagine the entire piece." Jamie's direction and choreography are never afterthoughts or something the artist does to fill in the spaces. It's all integral to the actual overall creative concept itself. Everything he has done, almost without exception, has been surprising and somehow has advanced pop culture. Jamie is the perfect person to have spent much of his working life with Madonna, because I haven't seen Jamie repeat himself yet. My hope for Jamie is that he doesn't quit. By definition, if he continues to be passionate and motivated, you know that he has surprises in store for us that we simply can't imagine.

Brian Graden is president of Entertainment, MTV Music Group, and president of Logo Network.

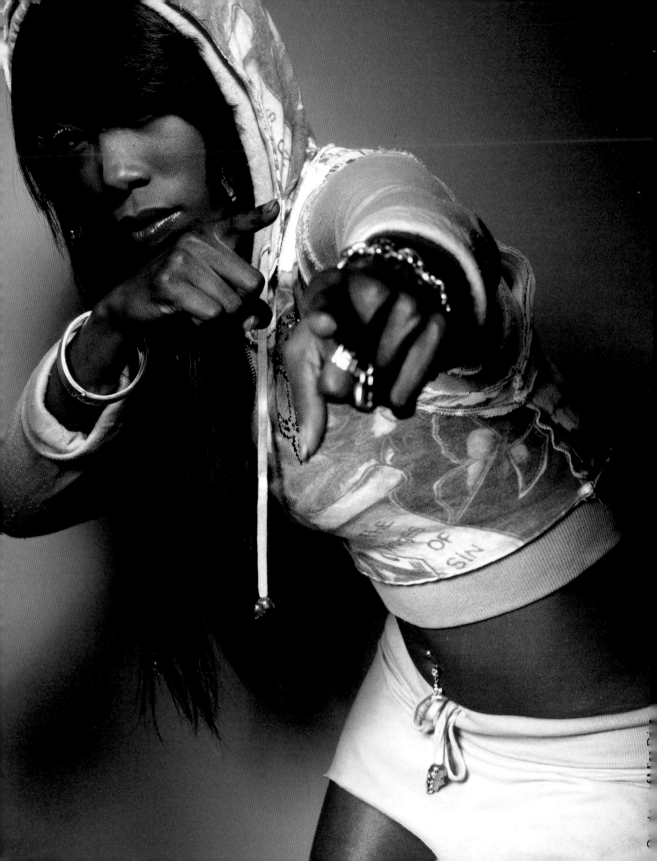

Miss Prissy

JAMIE ON MISS PRISSY: Miss Prissy was one of the star dancers in David LaChapelle's critically acclaimed dance documentary, *Rize*. Since then, she's worked with me on several projects, including Madonna's "Sorry" music video and tour, and has toured with Snoop Dogg and the Game. Her craft as a dancer is "extreme sport." Using her strength, her beauty, and her technical training, she's truly the "Queen of Krump."

MISS PRISSY ON JAMIE: My experience with Jamie was an eye-opener. I learned that being artistically expressive is very time consuming and requires a great deal of patience. Patience is so key in this business, and just being in Jamie's presence alone makes it rub off on you. He also taught me how to take my performances to another level—far past what I've ever expected. It heightened my senses of creativity. You just have to look at the stuff he had me doing in Madonna's "Sorry" video. Boy, did I learn my body that month.

Forget the "Perfect Body" Myth

Maybe you think you can't dance because you don't have a "perfect body." Get over it. There is no such thing as a perfect body. A perfect body is a body that feels healthy and fit. It's not a size 2 waist. It's a resting heart rate of 60, a cholesterol level below 120, a blood pressure of 120/80 or less.

I mean, look at someone like Nathan Lane, who starred in the Broadway musical (and then movie) *The Producers*. He's not a skinny guy. But he does a scene in that production in which he sings and dances in an almost continuous monologue in a small jail cell that, I kid you not, goes on for something like 14 minutes. It's the apogee of the entire show. The amount of stamina and fitness required for that kind of dancing has nothing to do with what size clothes you wear.

To me, Nathan Lane represents the embodiment of dance. Rent the movie and see what I mean. The absolute freedom with which he expresses himself is unbelievable. I guarantee that not only will you feel it yourself, but you will also want that same freedom for yourself.

While I'm on the topic, there's one other person I feel also embodies the spirit of dance without having the typical "dancer's" body. That's Ellen DeGeneres. You'd probably never think of her as a dancer, but she's the most perfect, amazing dancer I know. She's exactly the kind of dancer I want you to become. Why? Just watch her talk show one day.

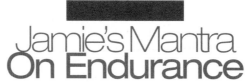

Jamie's Mantra
On Endurance

There are two types of endurance: physical endurance, which comes with practice and work; and mental endurance, which comes from within you. For instance, when I'm working on a tour with Madonna or Christina Aguilera, my mental endurance is constantly being tested. I have to be able to get by on very little sleep, manage a million little details, and still find room in it all for the creativity that will result in the unique movements themselves. But with every task completed, every tour under my belt, my mental endurance increases. Just as with every workout you complete, your physical endurance will increase.

How I Got Started

If you think getting started dancing is difficult for you, think about me. I was a kid growing up in a small town in Wisconsin, so you can just imagine the reactions of my parents, teachers, and friends when they found me dancing. I mean, in junior high I used to sit in front of MTV and write down the steps I saw the dancers doing so I could memorize them. How weird is that? But my mother, at least, finally "got it." In high school she gave me my own room in the basement that I decorated like a dance studio. I lived in that room—just me and my dog— making up dances. It took perseverance and grit to maintain my focus on my dream in the midst of the negativity around me, but I did it. And so can you!

On every show she has this little dance break. I just love watching it because it's the truest expression of dance you could ever capture. It's so infectious that everyone who sees her wants to get up there and dance with her. Just with that little dance break she inspires a world. It's the same thing I've been trying to do for years.

Another good example is Missy Elliott. I mean, she's the highest-selling female rapper of all time, dominating the rap industry, and she dances her heart out. But she's not some anorexic model.

And that's the point. Whether you're *zaftig*—plump and sexy—or you're super-model size because you can't gain weight and that's just your body type, as long as you can move, you can dance.

Set Your Rockin' Goals

Here's something I promise you: Once you master Rock Your Body, you'll feel empowered beyond the dance, able to take on things you didn't know you could handle. Because finding success in one part of your life invariably leads to success in others.

Which brings me to goal setting.

As you go through the Rock Your Body workout, I want you to think of it as more than just a workout. It's a door opening to your dreams—even if those dreams have nothing to do with dance. Because by taking this first risk—trying something new, something you didn't think you could do—you're opening yourself up for other risks.

And forget about all the people in your life who tell you that your dream is ridiculous or unachievable. If I'd listened to everyone who told me I'd never be a famous choreographer/director, I'd probably be grilling hamburgers right now. Instead, every time someone told me "no," or "not happening," or to give up, it just made me fight harder. That's why I urge everyone I know—especially you—to constantly reach higher, ask for more, and never give up—even if it seems too difficult. Push yourself and keep going . . . I promise that extra push will bring real rewards.

For instance, if you thought you could never dance, and now you find yourself whipping through both Rock Your Body routines with no problem, then what's to keep you from getting that real estate license you've been talking about? Losing those last 10 pounds? Running that marathon? Remember the promotion at work your friend told you to go for, but you were too afraid of failing to even apply? Well, it's time to get moving.

But don't rely only on long-term goals. I want to see you setting some short-term goals, too. For instance, one goal could be to have the Rock Your Body routine down by Christmas.

And make your goals concrete. I get so tired of hearing people say all the time, "One day I'm going to do *this*," and "One day I'm going to do *that*." Listen, the "one day" is now, it's today. You don't get another day. So if you keep putting off the idea of getting your body in shape, of starting the Rock Your Body routine, you're never going to get to where you want to be—in anything.

To help you in setting your goals, I've provided a goal-setting worksheet. Fill it in, then check off each goal as you reach it.

Carrie Ann Inaba

JAMIE ON CARRIE ANN:

If anyone knows dance, it's Carrie Ann Inaba, one of three judges on ABC's hit show *Dancing with the Stars*. Carrie Ann is not only a judge on DWTS, but she's also a terrific choreographer and my personal friend. She's also choreographed numerous television events, including *American Idol* Christmas 2003, *Miss America* 1998–2001 and 2003, *All-American Girl* 2003, and *Who Wants to Marry a Millionaire*, and acted and danced in films and television series including *In Living Color, Showgirls,* and *Flintstones 2: Viva Rock Vegas!*

CARRIE ANN ON JAMIE:

I think Jamie's vision is "sensual." In his shows for Madonna and other stars, he creates a wonderful fantasy world. He has a fantastic fashion sense, which touches every aspect of his productions. When you watch them, you feel like you are inside a complete landscape. I respect him enormously for the amount of research he does for his work. It makes a huge difference in every project he takes on. That's why his workout will be so successful: I'm sure he spent hours developing it. He inspires many people. He'll inspire anyone who does his workout.

Jamie's Mantra
On Perseverance

One of my favorite dance movies is *Flashdance*. Not just because of the amazing dancing and choreography in the movie. But also because of the storyline. It's a story about perseverance. About not being technically trained and having a great fear, but of pushing through that fear. I've had to do it. I've had times when I was younger when I'd go to an audition and leave because I felt intimidated, but I'd force myself to go back and conquer that fear and not give in. And that's just what I want you to do.

And be flexible. If your goal is to have the whole Rock Your Body routine down within 2 weeks and you get the flu, don't just chuck it all. Simply readjust your goal.

In the next chapter I'll show you how to find the motivation you need to reach your goals.

Goal Worksheet

Goal	Steps required	Estimated time to completion	Step completed	Goal obtained
My goal is to . . .	1.			
	2.			
	3.			
	4.			
My goal is to . . .				
My goal is to . . .				
My goal is to . . .				
My goal is to . . .				
My goal is to . . .				
My goal is to . . .				
My goal is to . . .				

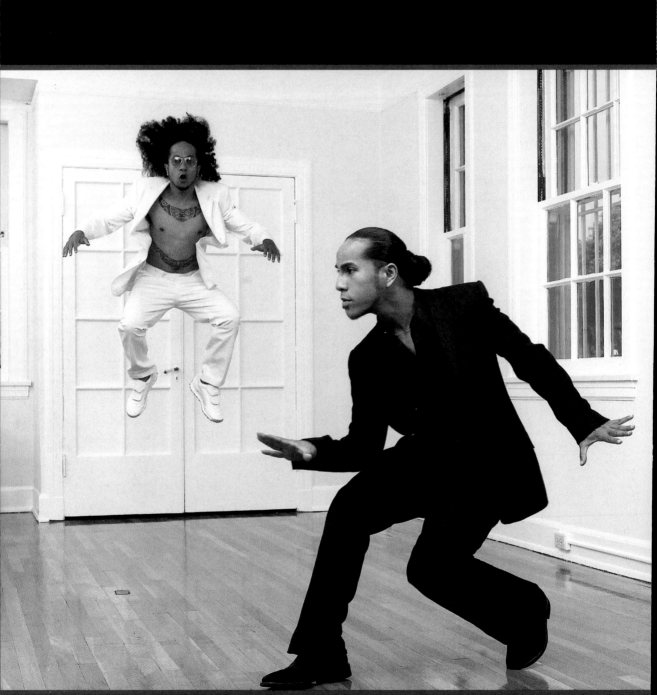

Acclaimed Choreographers
Richmond and Tone Talauega

RICHMOND ON JAMIE: I think dance is a great way to get and stay fit. Reason being is because dancing works almost every muscle in the body. The synergy between rhythm and coordination done to a steady beat (music, if needed) is cardiovascular. It's exercising, but with graceful movement. A personal benefit I get from dance that I love is *balance.* Dance is an ancient form of communication. I communicate my emotions through dance, like aggression, love, confidence, etc. It brings me to a state of humbleness. What sets Jamie King apart from other directors that I worked with is his creative style of adapting. For the plethora of artists that he works with, each has had their own distinct vibe. He has an instinct for knowing what artists need and what people want to see. Jamie King is a Scientist of Pop Culture.

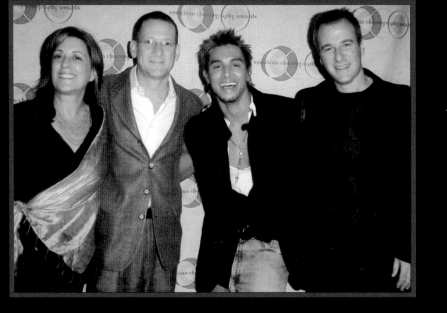

Left to right: Agent Julie McDonald, producer/manager Daniel Sladek, American Choreography Award nominee Jamie King, and agent Tony Selznick at the American Choreography Awards in Los Angeles

Tony Selznick

JAMIE ON TONY: Tony Selznick has been my agent for more than 10 years and comes from a dance background himself.

TONY ON JAMIE: Jamie is one of those people that makes you want to work hard. His sense of motivation and self is so strong that he constantly makes you want to be your best always. He has the quintessential qualities of any good director or producer: incredible leadership and the ability to make you feel important in the world. But what I love most about him is that he's very honest and he says what's on his mind all the time. You can always rely on him for that. So trust Jamie. If you don't trust your teachers, you won't learn anything from them."

Julie McDonald

JAMIE ON JULIE: When her own dance career was cut short by injury, Julie McDonald formed the first talent agency to represent dancers and choreographers. She, along with her partner, Tony Selznick, has been my agent for more than a decade. Here she talks about the first time she saw my Nike Rockstar Workout in a Hollywood club.

JULIE ON JAMIE: I walked away feeling that the production represented a level so high and so good it would challenge everyone in the field. Jamie has such a great vision about how things should be and how to bring it to fruition. He's a conceptual artist, and even though he may not do every step himself, he knows what it should look like. I think he's raised the level of commercial dance to something other directors and choreographers aspire to achieve.

Reach higher.
Ask for **more.**
Never give up.

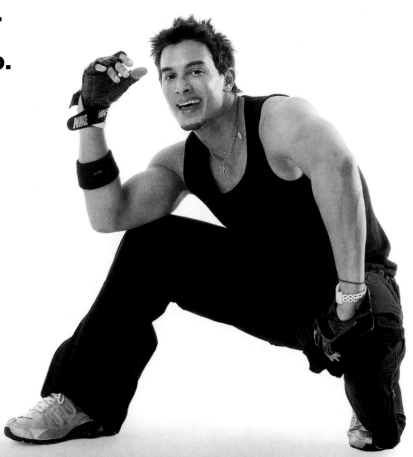

Chapter 3
Rock Your Mind

Despite all the fabulous things I've told you about the benefits of dance, it wouldn't surprise me if you're still struggling with the "m" word: motivation. Or maybe you've gone through the Rock Your Body workout a few times but now find yourself making excuses for avoiding it. You're too busy. You have a cold. Your kid is sick. Your dog needs to go to the vet.

Hey, we've all been there. I can't tell you how many performers I work with who can take to the stage and belt out a song with no problem. But when I tell them they have to move and dance, they're terrified. I had this very situation with Ricky Martin when I first started working with him.

Here's a performer who spent much of the early years of his career focused on dancing and choreography. But when he hired me to artistically guide his career in a new direction, he wasn't sure he wanted dance to be a part of it. I think he was just tired of the steps and choreography and rigidness of what he'd previously known as "dance." It seemed to me that he'd lost his motivation to dance.

From the beginning, however, I knew we couldn't rule out dance. It was as if we really didn't have a choice, given the musicality and infectious nature of his music. You simply *had* to dance to that sound! Yet he kept telling me he was at a place in his career where he wanted to have fun. And dance, he felt, didn't offer him that opportunity.

Jamie's Mantra
On a Positive Attitude

A positive attitude is the key to success and to living a great life. For instance, if I hadn't been positive that I could get a job dancing for Prince when I was still a teenager, I wouldn't have risked being kicked out of dance school by auditioning. I got the job and it launched my professional career. Resist self-judgment and judgment from others.

I knew immediately he'd never really learned the true nature of dance. "Let's explore what dance really is," I said. "Let's not worry about choreography and step one and step two and step three. Let's just explore what the music tells our bodies and make that our choreography."

So instead of turning dance into a rigid formula he had to learn, we let it become an expression of himself. His motivation returned. And so will yours. First, though, you have to ask yourself one important question: Are you ready to change your life and allow dance into it?

Getting Ready to Change

Whether it's starting an exercise program, quitting smoking, cutting up the credit cards, or giving up a bad relationship, change is hard. You don't just wake up one morning and decide to change. Instead, I've learned, you go through a process, one called the Stages of Change.

This process has been studied in all kinds of behavior changes, including exercise and diet. It's a process, however, not an end to itself. What I mean by that is that even though you've completed one stage and moved on to another, there's always the possibility that you'll return to that earlier stage.

Here are the five Stages of Change. Which stage are you currently in?

1. **Precontemplation stage.** In this stage you haven't even begun to think about changing. If you're overweight and a couch potato, you tell yourself that you like

yourself this way. You're in denial about health problems and the need to change. I'm betting most of you are beyond this stage, however, since you've already purchased *Rock Your Body.*

2. **Contemplation stage.** In this stage you've started thinking about changing but aren't quite sure it's a step you really want to take. On the one hand you like the idea of incorporating a fitness program like Rock Your Body into your life; but on the other hand, you don't think you have enough time or energy for it, and you wonder what you'll have to give up to carve out the time and energy. Some of you are probably in this stage, which is why you're reading this book.

3. **Preparation stage.** Okay, in this stage you've decided it's time for a change. You decide you're going to get in shape. You might start taking small steps now. Like purchasing a fitness book. Or walking for 10 minutes a day. Or buying some exercise clothes.

4. **Action stage.** You'll know you've reached this stage when you start doing the Rock Your Body workout. Give yourself a big pat on the back. This is a big moment in your life, and one you should be really proud of.

5. **Maintenance and relapse prevention.** This is the hard part of the Stages of Change—maintaining that action stage and preventing yourself from relapsing into your old couch potato habits. Oh, sure, it's easy when you first start doing the workout, when you're having fun, releasing endorphins, feeling sexy. You start to feel alive and invigorated. But once that feeling becomes routine, how do you keep motivating yourself?

One way is by not letting a small relapse become a big one. Say you miss a week because you're on vacation. That's okay! Your muscles have retained the memory of the Rock Your Body workout. Just start up again, and within a session or two, you'll be right back where you left off. This is the same philosophy that says don't give up on your healthy way of eating just because you had one junk-food-filled weekend!

The bottom line is that no one can motivate you but *you*. If you want to succeed, if you want to be great at this workout, then you have to motivate yourself. So don't sit around waiting for someone else to come up, clap you on the back, and beg you to get out your *Rock Your Body* book and start working out. That can only come from within you.

(continued)

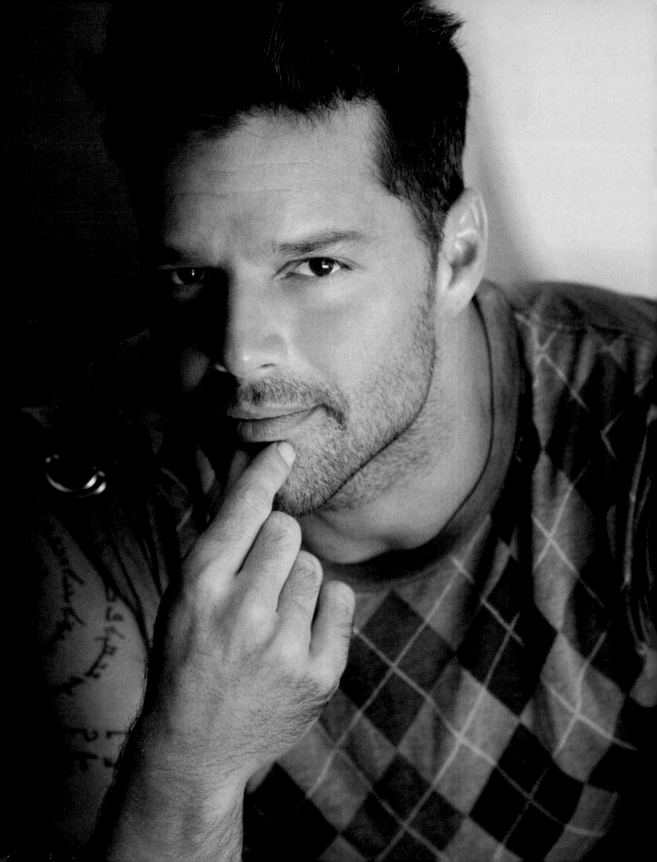

Ricky Martin

JAMIE ON RICKY: I directed Ricky's *Livin' La Vida Loca* and *Black and White* world tours. He may not have been technically trained but he dances from his heart with passion and soul, and he taught the world how to "shake their hips." That rocks!

RICKY ON JAMIE: Since I first worked with Jamie on my *Livin' La Vida Loca* world tour in 1999, I was amazed by his talent and creativity. His innovative technique, mixing dance moves with fitness, has been key in all of my productions, and I have continued to use it throughout the years. In my opnion, he has created a new and effective way to take the show to a different level. Even though my moves on stage are innate, Jamie helps bring out the best in me.

Here's what my personal trainer Omar Lopez recommends for motivation: "Be fully present and get rid of all your distractions," he says. "Only think about what you are doing. And try not to be so attached to results. You'll be amazed at how freeing and energizing it is."

Omar calls this internal motivation "clearness." I call it desire. I see it every day in the dancers and rock stars I work with. I see it in the young dancer who dances even though his feet are bleeding. I see it in the rock star who attends 10-hour rehearsals to prepare for another tour even though she doesn't need the money from the tour or the additional fame it will bring. I see it in the dancer-turned-choreographer who is

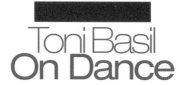

Toni Basil
On Dance

Toni Basil is one of the top choreographers in show business. She choreographed Legally Blonde, My Best Friend's Wedding *and* American Graffiti. *She created shows and videos for Enrique Iglesias, Paris Hilton, The Pussycat Dolls, Tina Turner, Mick Jagger, David Bowie, and Bette Midler, with whom she works regularly. As an original member of the break-dancing group The Lockers, she is credited with popularizing street dance, thereby revolutionizing contemporary dance. And we all know the lyrics to her hit song: "Oh Mickey, you're so fine . . . " Here are her thoughts on dance.*

"Motivation is the most important element for a dancer. Body type doesn't matter. If you start out like I did, the passion grows into an addiction. Even the stars don't have to be great dancers. In fact, a lot of them can't dance. But their physical movement has to support the music. Look at Steve Tyler of Aerosmith. He's not a dancer but he hits every beat. He gives a really visual performance."

As for herself, she says: "I'm obsessive in a creative way. When I'm dancing and choreographing, I get a buzz. I don't notice anything. I'm not aware of obstacles, only of doing what I love. I was lucky enough to grow up in show business with my mother, a comedic, acrobatic dancer, and my father, an orchestra conductor. So dance is in my blood. I can't recall ever not dancing around the house."

scared to death of taking this next step but who has a fierce desire within himself to create—and knows this is the only way to get there.

You're not alone in your struggle with motivation. My friend and fellow choreographer Mia Michaels says she battles with it every day. "Although I've always been very, very focused and very clear about my career, and never had a problem with motivation for my career, I'm only beginning to understand the need to stay motivated about my physical self." At 40, she says, she's finally begun to understand that every day is a gift and another chance to make herself feel healthier and more alive.

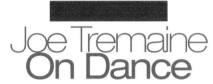

Joe Tremaine On Dance

Joe Tremaine played a crucial role in my life when he awarded me a scholarship to his dance school in Los Angeles when I was a teenager. Embarking on the 26th year of Tremaine Dance Convention and Competitions, Joe remains one of the most influential dance personalities in the country today. He is an internationally known choreographer, teacher, and performer, having worked with Cameron Diaz, Christina Applegate, Academy-Award winner Helen Hunt, Goldie Hawn, Jamie Lee Curtis, Diana Ross, Jerry Lewis, and Regis Philbin, to name just a few. In April 2001 he received a lifetime achievement award from the Palm Desert California Dance Under the Stars concert series. His motto is, "Let's dance for health and happiness." Here are his thoughts on dance.

"What you need to succeed in dance is dedication—the kind of dedication Jamie has. You also need technique and to get training. That's hardly the whole thing, but it gives you a good foundation. I always tell kids to get as much dance education as possible—not just ballet, jazz, tap, and hip-hop, but flamenco and Cuban-American, whatever is available. Just look at how Jamie fuses many styles in his work.

"To succeed you also need passion. You can't let anyone stop you. The most challenging part of this world is the competition. A young woman might show up for an audition and there will be 500 others wanting the same job. Jamie went through that just like every other dancer who comes to Los Angeles."

But having the desire alone isn't enough. You also have to have a commitment to turn that desire into action. So, for instance, if your desire is to tone your body, the steps necessary to turn that desire into action might be:

1. Decide on a fitness routine.
2. Join the gym . . . schedule the class . . . buy the book or DVD . . . for that particular fitness regimen.
3. Complete the first workout.
4. Go back again and again until the fitness routine has become as much a part of your life as brushing your teeth.
5. Check out your body. Have you accomplished your desire?

I know that whenever you take on anything new, it can be scary. And I know a lot of people are scared of change because it's uncomfortable. But listen: I want you to take that fear and that uncomfortable feeling and turn it into a strength. You should be excited about being uncomfortable! You know what I'm saying? Comfort is boring. The second you start to feel comfortable—like if the workout starts to become easy—that's when you need to be scared. That's when you need to punch everything up a

Christina Aguilera
On Dance

Not only has dance been a form of expression and a creative outlet for me, but it also has been a key exercise tool to help me stay fit and in shape for all the other elements that go into my work. Plus I think it is necessary that women in particular get enough exercise in our lives because heart disease continues to be the leading cause of death in women. Having said that, it's important that we all find a fun and inventive way of staying in shape, and I can't think of a better way than dance. Not only do you get a sense of accomplishment by mastering a dance move or routine, but dance also helps build stamina through its cardiovascular elements and provides more energy thoughout the day in all facets of whatever you do.

notch. Because that means you're at the stage where life could easily pass by you.

So it's perfectly normal to be terrified of starting this new fitness routine, of how losing weight and toning your body will affect your life, change your relationships. That's great! It means you're going to learn from it. You're going to learn something new about yourself and what you can accomplish—things you thought you'd never be able to accomplish.

And do you know the only way to get comfortable doing something you're not comfortable with?

Do it!

And do it over and over again. Train, study, conquer it! Conquer the fear!

I promise you that the more you do something, the more you'll want to do it and the less you'll worry about your motivation. Think about when you get into the car. Do you have to actually remember to put on your seat belt, or do you do it automatically as you take a breath?

How many times have you been in the shower and you can't remember if you've washed your hair because it's so automatic? You've built up muscle memory in your brain. And the same thing will happen with Rock Your Body. After a few weeks of this workout, especially once you see your inner dancer's body emerge, you'll find that if you try to skip a day you feel strange. Weird. Like something's off. Because your muscle memory wants to know—hey, dude, where's the workout for the day?

Robin Antin

JAMIE ON ROBIN: One of the most highly respected choreographers in show business, Robin has incorporated her innate passion for the art of dance and her deeply rooted drive into a long roster of top-quality projects for stars such as Sting, Pink, Ricky Martin, and No Doubt. She choreographed *The Sweetest Thing, View from the Top,* and *Charlie's Angels,* and the MTV Movie Awards. She created the all-female burlesque group The Pussycat Dolls in 1993, which now includes a Las Vegas nightclub venue and floorshow and a reality TV series. I consider her responsible for bringing back burlesque.

ROBIN ON JAMIE: Jamie has a super creative mind. He's inspired by a diverse array of music, dance, and photography. You can see it in his choreography, which is like no one else's. When I worked with him with The Smashing Pumpkins for the American Music Awards, I found out he's a complete perfectionist. He knows directing and choreographing inside out and comes to a project knowing exactly what he wants to achieve.

What Jamie has done with Madonna is amazing. He's had an incredible effect on pop culture through her. He can reach the widest demographics because of his wide-ranging interests. I love his masculine vibe. Even when he choreographs for women, he keeps that masculine feel. That's why his becoming Nike's dance-as-sport representative makes absolute sense. His dancers have the force and energy of the most competitive sports.

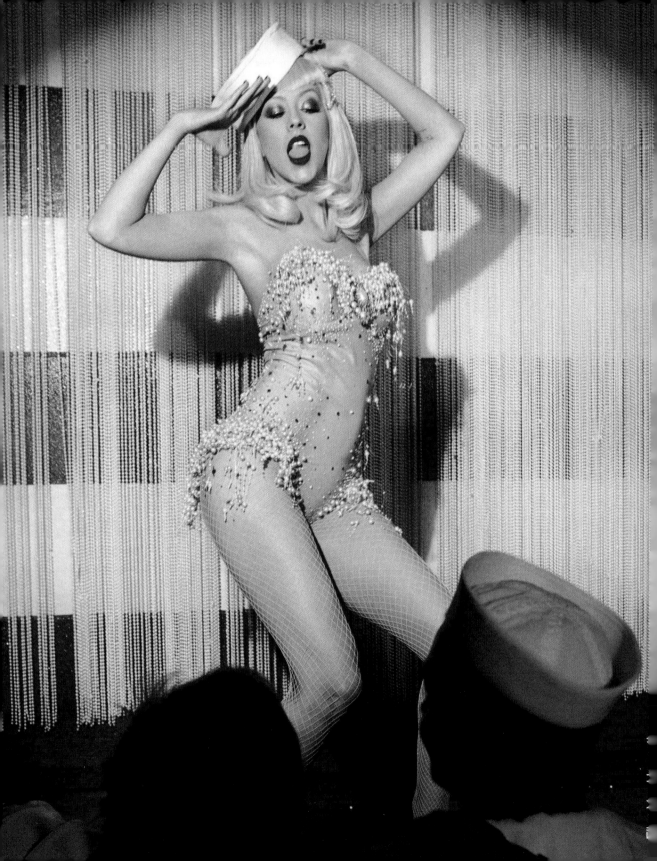

Christina Aguilera

JAMIE ON CHRISTINA: I directed Christina's *Stripped* and *Back to Basics* world tours. She is a performer who has just persevered. She's had to struggle through a lot to get where she is now, and she had to have a strong conviction as a woman in this business to get where she is. As for dance . . . she's got great style. Vampy and sexy. When she moves, it's her own unique style. Just great. And best of all: She fights for what she believes in.

CHRISTINA ON JAMIE: Working with Jamie is always a fun, new, and exciting journey each and every time. His creativity and attention to details is refreshing and inspiring. He has a true knack for getting inside an artist's head and understanding their vision, tapping into a whole new world of imagination for both the performers and audience alike to enjoy.

Part II
Rock Your Body Workout

If you run into the wall,
slide down it
and **make it**
look sexy!

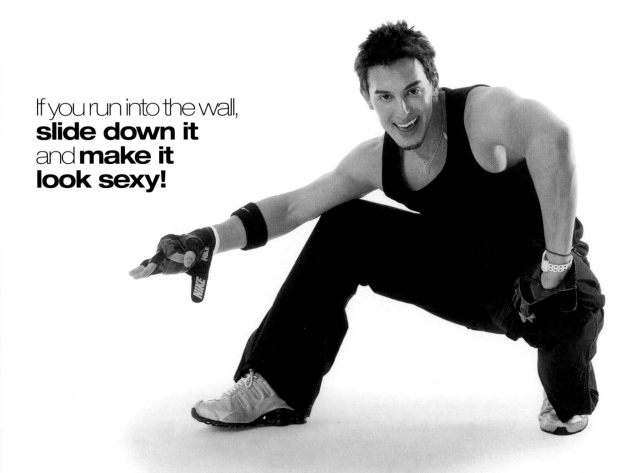

Chapter 4
Time to Rock!

So now we come to the part you've been waiting for: the actual Rock Your Body program. And now I can answer the question I'm sure you've all been asking: Is it really possible to learn to dance from a book? And just as important: Is it possible to get a sexy body from a book?

Absolutely! In my mind, getting a sexy body is 50 percent mental, 30 percent conditioning, and 20 percent dedication.

Listen, many of the dancers and stars I work with, like Ricky Martin and Ellen DeGeneres, never had any formal dance training. They came to it the way you're coming to it—on their own. That's really how I learned to dance, you know—I taught myself. I copied things off the TV until I was able to get into a dance class. I practiced in my bedroom. And I didn't even have a mirror in which to watch myself.

You can do it, too!

But like anything else in life, it takes practice. You can't just try the Rock Your Body workout and decide it's too difficult. You have to stick with it. One of the best ways to integrate it into your daily life is to start slow. Work on two or three moves a day until you feel you've got them down perfectly. The next day, move on to the next three moves. It may take a couple of weeks before you're rocking the entire routine, but that's okay! No one is watching, no one is judging, no one is evaluating.

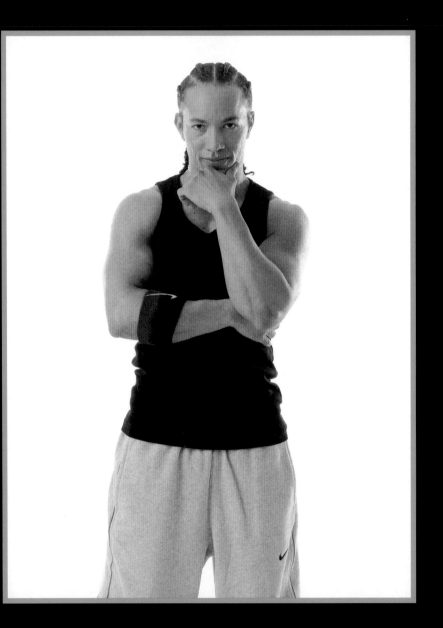

Celebrity trainer Omar Lopez

The beauty of this approach is that you're slowly building up your core—your abdomen, back muscles, butt. All your strength and all the moves in the routine begin and end with the core. And even if it takes you 6 months to finally get to the point where you can work your way through the entire Rock Your Body program, including both routines, I guarantee it won't take nearly that long before you begin seeing the benefits in your body.

For instance, one of the moves I have you do involves leaning your chest back and your hips forward. That move looks really simple, but it's hard work that requires deep control from within your core. This is the kind of work that will really show up on your body.

As my personal trainer Omar Lopez says: "Core strength is especially helpful to dancers, who need it for balance, flexibility, and stability."

Overall, through the Rock Your Body program you're getting the same kind of workout you'd get in a gym or running around the track—only more. Not only are you getting the cardio training, but you're also building your endurance and muscle tone and definition at the same time. But most important, you're doing it while having fun!

If you don't believe me, maybe you'll believe Omar. I heard about him through dancers in Los Angeles who had worked with him on tour with Janet Jackson. They raved about the extent of his knowledge of the body and his amazing way of getting the most out of clients. He's worked with Mary J. Blige, Prince, Madonna, P Diddy, and Usher. It also helps that he is one of the most thoughtful and patient men I know.

Omar also has his own dance background, which is how he came to fitness. "When I was dancing with Janet Jackson, I heard about her trainer Douglas Yee and saw the result of his work with Janet," he recalls. "A couple of the other dancers had started using his fitness techniques, and it definitely gave them an edge. They became more than just good performers. That's what started me seriously paying attention to what it means to be fit and well conditioned."

Omar considers his dance background priceless. "It's made me coordinated, helped me understand how my body works, and given me enormous confidence on and off the stage."

Two Core Exercises

I asked Omar to give me a couple of exercises that work for the core.
Here are two he recommends:

The Bridge: Lie on your back with your knees bent and slowly lift your pelvis up and down a few times with your arms at your sides.

The Plank: Lie on your stomach and raise yourself up on your elbows, pulling your navel into your spine to stretch the lower back and keeping your legs on the floor. Still facing the floor, raise yourself up on your elbows and toes, keeping your back flat and your stomach in. Hold the position for 30 seconds. Relax, then repeat.

The best way to get and stay fit, he says, is to find something you like so you'll stick with it. "That's why dancing is so great. Most people love to dance once they get over their self-consciousness. And you can do it almost anywhere."

Even if you're not dancing, however, he advises getting some kind of exercise every day. "It can be taking a walk, using the stairs instead of an elevator, or dancing around your living room," Omar says. "Of course, an organized workout will do you more good, but the most important thing is to move, use your muscles, and exert yourself. No question, it will always make you feel better and more alive."

As you ready yourself to begin the Rock Your Body workout, keep in mind something else Omar taught me: The most important thing in becoming fit is your alignment, or posture. "It's your foundation," he explains. "If you're not aligned correctly, your body will compensate and you'll wear down your muscles and joints." That's why the first thing he does when he starts with a new client is put him or her in the correct position. If you can't position yourself correctly, he says, "get a trainer or someone familiar with physical training to put you in the cor-

Celebrities I've Worked With: Janet Jackson

Janet is a badass dancer. She's defined dance for the last two decades and is a true inspiration. When I was younger, I used to copy her moves from her music videos. When I was on break from touring with her brother Michael, she asked me to dance in her music video "If." That was a dream come true.

rect position for your body. Memorize it and catch yourself when you slip out of it."

Julie Daugherty, physical therapist for the American Ballet Theater, also believes in the importance of good posture. "Many people sit at desks all day, with their heads down and their shoulders slouched forward, which can lead to back and neck problems. The good posture required when you dance is a great way to counteract the problems that can arise from a sedentary lifestyle."

Let me say one other thing: When you watch a performer like Madonna on the stage, she makes it seem so easy, as if she just decided to jump up there and move her body however the music moves her. What you're not seeing are the 6 months of 14-hour rehearsals, day in and day out, when she's had to learn every step and repeat it and repeat it and repeat it.

Matthew Rolston

JAMIE ON MATTHEW:

Matthew Rolston is one of the best music video directors and photographers I've ever worked with. He's brought his eye for classic composition and style to some of the top performers in the industry—including Madonna, Janet Jackson, David Bowie, and Beyonce Knowles.

MATTHEW ON JAMIE:

There's a special fire that burns hot and bright inside everything Jamie King creates. There's always an exciting presentness . . . an attitude of tension and intensity in his choreography.

How Fit Are You?

Before you begin the workout, let's talk a bit about your own fitness level. Do you do something athletic every day? Or do you consider workouts best reserved for the category of "Things We Do Not Discuss," like religion, sex, and politics? It really doesn't matter; with a little work and time, the Rock Your Body workout will become your own.

Nonetheless, knowing where you're starting from will help you determine how to approach the workout. It will also give you a baseline from which to track your progress. So I want you to answer the following questions—and be honest. If you're not honest, you know, you're only hurting yourself. Then retake the quiz after 4 weeks of Rock Your Body workouts. You'll be amazed at the difference.

Rock Your Body Fitness Analysis

Health Indication	Response (circle one)	Advice
I sleep well at night . . .	Always Sometimes I know every joke Conan O'Brien has told for the past 10 years.	Forget the bags under your eyes. If you're not sleeping well, you're putting yourself at risk for a host of health problems, including diabetes, obesity, and depression. No worries, though; the regular exercise you'll get through the Rock Your Body workout should help with any insomnia.
My body recovers easily from injuries . . .	Almost always Sometimes I keep the number for the ER on speed dial.	If your body takes a while to recover from injuries like scrapes or sprains, you could have a weak immune system. Following a sensible diet and getting regular physical activity should help boost your immune system.
I get colds, flu, stomach viruses, and other infections . . .	Never Sometimes I keep my doctor's home number on speed dial.	See above
I eat fast food . . .	Never Once or twice a month Every time I pass the Golden Arches.	Here's the thing: Every time you swing by the drive-thru, along with your burger and fries you're also getting dangerously high amounts of calories, fat, saturated fat, and salt. This is one habit you've got to break. So listen: Follow the Dancer's Diet Commandments for 2 weeks and don't eat any junk food during that time. After 2 weeks, your taste buds will have changed and I guarantee that burger will have lost its appeal.
I get ___ servings of fruit and vegetables a day most days.	1–3 I'm nearly a vegetarian Do French fries count?	No, French fries don't count (neither does red wine). If you're low on fruit and veggies, you're missing out on valuable cancer-fighting phytonutrients, not to mention weight-reducing fiber. In fact, estimates are that as many as 20 percent of all cancers could be prevented if people just ate more fruit and veggies. The Dancer's Diet shows you how to incorporate more of these foods into your meals.
I eat red meat . . .	Rarely 1–3 times a week Is there any other kind?	Keep eating that red meat and you're putting yourself at serious risk for pancreatic and colon cancer. If you must eat red meat, aim for the leanest you can find. Wild game is a good choice, as are certain cuts of beef and pork.

Rock Your Body Fitness Analysis

Health Indication	Response (circle one)	Advice
I smoke . . .	Yes (but I'm trying to quit, I swear) Only in bars Can't stand the stuff	With few exceptions, I don't think anyone *chooses* to smoke. And I understand that smoking is an addiction. So don't try to quit on your own. Get your doctor involved. There are drugs, patches, gums, and candies designed to wean you off nicotine and into a healthier life.
I drink alcohol . . .	It's still Prohibition in my house 1–2 times a week Whenever the clock strikes 5:00 p.m. (somewhere in the world)	Hey, I'm not a teetotaler. But if you're quaffing more than one or two a day—especially if you're a woman—you're putting yourself at risk for a whole host of problems, including breast cancer, liver disease, and high blood pressure. So follow my mantra: Everything in moderation.
I drink something caffeinated . . .	Never 1–2 times a day I'm a preferred member at Starbucks	To be honest, I think the negatives of caffeine have been strongly overrated. Heck, there's even some evidence coffee drinkers are less likely to get diabetes! But if you're having trouble sleeping at night, then it's time to cut back, or at the very least, turn off the caffeine spigot after 2:00 p.m.
I drink water . . .	With my scotch When I'm thirsty Throughout the day	As you'll see in the Dancer's Diet on page 175, I'm a big proponent of drinking water—lots of water. It helps clear toxins from your body, helps your skin stay young and fresh looking, and keeps hunger at bay. So grab a bottle (or three or four) whenever you head out the door or even to your desk.
When bad things happen I . . .	Tend to look on the bright side Hide under my covers	I'm a firm believer in the proverbial "look on the bright side" philosophy. No matter what happens, good or bad, I believe it happens for a reason. So instead of focusing on the negative, I find the positive. Turns out this kind of thinking actually makes me healthier by helping me manage stress better. So I highly recommend you try it. Here's one example: You're stuck in traffic and you're late to a meeting. You can get all steamed and do terrible things to your body, or you can accept that you are powerless over the traffic, but that you have power over your reaction and how you spend your time in traffic. Call a friend you haven't spoken to for a while, put on your favorite CD and belt out a song, make up a to-do list. Suddenly, that traffic jam isn't such a terrible thing, is it?

(continued)

Rock Your Body Fitness Analysis —*Continued*

Health Indication	Response (circle one)	Advice
My weight is . . .	Just fine Rising faster than ticket prices for rock concerts	You can be "overweight" and still be in shape. And in the scheme of things, I'm going to put being in shape as the most important thing. But as you know by now, dancing through the Rock Your Body workout three or four times a week, along with following the Dancer's Diet Commands, should peel the pounds right off. At the very least, I promise you're going to be much happier with the way your body looks—no matter what the scale says.
I'm so flexible I can . . .	Touch my toes without bending my knees Sit in a chair—sometimes	Ah, babies. They're so flexible they can suck their own toes. While I do know a few super-flexible dancers who could probably do that, for most of us that level of flexibility is gone forever. Nonetheless, the Rock Your Body workout will improve your overall flexibility. Why is this important? Because the more flexible you are, the better your muscles and joints move, reducing the risk of injury. The more flexible you are, the less likely you are to have lower back pain, a stiff neck, shoulder pain. Just wait— check your flexibility again in about 4 weeks and tell me where you are. I guarantee your whole body will feel looser and more "stretched out."
I try to work out . . .	Every time there's a presidential election Every time there's a full moon Four or five times a week	If you're already working out on a regular basis (I try to get an hour workout in every day when I can), then you're 10 steps ahead of the crowd. The Rock Your Body workout will bring your workout to an entirely new dimension. But if you're new to working out, take it slow. You may not want to start with the entire workout at once. And do me a favor: Check with your doctor before you begin the program. Rock Your Body is fairly strenuous, and I want to make sure you can handle it.
My stress level is . . .	Only a problem when my mother visits The reason I go through a bottle of antacids a week	If you have a low stress level, you're either living in a beach hut in Bali or you're drinking too much. No, seriously, most of us wouldn't know what a stress-free life feels like. And I'm not going to tell you that the Rock Your Body workout will get rid of stress in your life. What it *will* do, however, is help you better manage your stress so it doesn't do you in. Return to Chapter 1 and reread the section on stress.

Making Rock Your Body Your Own

There are two ways to do the Rock Your Body program: the right way and the wrong way. The wrong way is to view it as a series of exercises that happen to look like dancing, exercises you must follow to the letter. Exercises that will eventually get pretty boring.

The right way is to make the program your own. Here's what I mean. When I work with my rock stars, I don't impose a style on them. I don't go to Ricky Martin or Christina Aguilera and say, "Here's what you should do," because it's what *I* want them to do. No. I develop everything from the choreography to the music to the lighting based on that individual and what he or she has to say, the persona they're trying to project. My goal is to come up with something that really works *for them,* so *they* feel and look their best.

And that's exactly what I've done with the Rock Your Body workout. This workout is designed to be flexible enough to allow you to change it if you want, strong enough to give you the intense fitness workout you're looking for, and intense enough to challenge you to reach new levels you didn't know you could even aim for.

It's designed to make you feel great about doing something you haven't done before, to make you feel excited that you're doing something fresh. It's designed to rock your mind, body, and soul. And most important—it's designed to make sure you have *fun.* Because really, if you're not having fun, what's the point?

Rock Your Body is also designed as a modular program so you can mix and match the parts. Here's how they break out timewise:

Warmup: 10 minutes
Strength training: 10 minutes
Rock Your Body Routine 1: 15 minutes
Rock Your Body Routine 2: 15 minutes
Cooldown: 2 minutes

So here are a few ways you could put together the parts:

- Warmup + Routine 1 + Cooldown (27 minutes)
- Warmup + Strength training + Cooldown (22 minutes)
- Warmup + Routine 2 + Cooldown (27 minutes)
- Warmup + Routine 1 + Routine 2 + Cooldown (42 minutes)
- Warmup + Strength training + Routine 1 + Cooldown (37 minutes)
- Warmup + Strength training + Routine 2 + Cooldown (37 minutes)

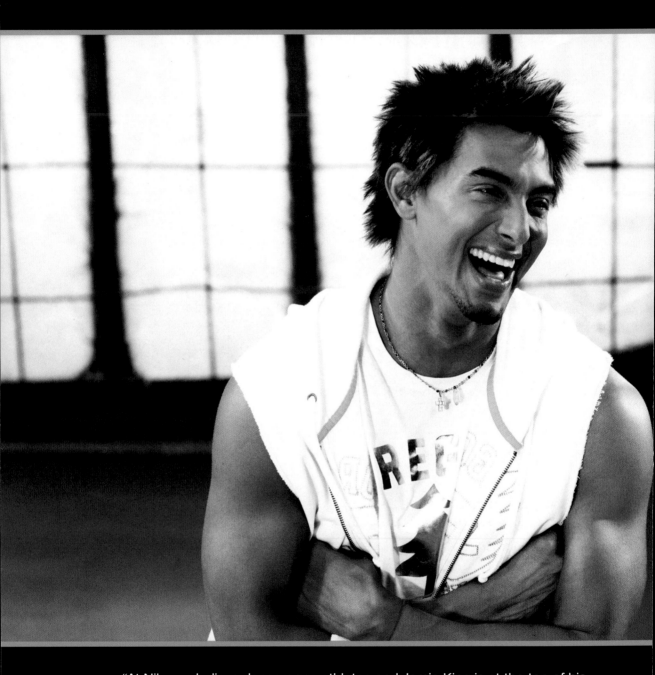

"At Nike we believe dancers are athletes and Jamie King is at the top of his game. When you consider the rhythm, agility, balance, energy, grace, and stamina it takes to be a success in dance, you appreciate like we do what Jamie has accomplished. Jamie has been a valuable partner to Nike in helping us to draw attention to and innovate in the fitness dance category."
—Darcy Winslow, Global Women's Fitness Director, NIKE

The full workout, warmup plus strength training plus Routine 1 plus Routine 2 plus cooldown, will give you a fantastic 52-minute workout, about an hour with breaks.

This flexibility is ideal because we both know that there will be times when you simply can't fit the entire workout into your day. All I ask is that even on those days, you do at least one or two parts. I guarantee it will improve the quality of your day, no matter how stressful it's been.

Feeling Your Inner Rock Star

If you're used to thinking of dance as a series of learned steps that must be accompanied by music, then you're not thinking of dance in the right way. Sure, the centerpiece of Rock Your Body is a carefully choreographed set of steps and movements designed to tone and tighten your body, but that's just one aspect of dance. Dance, in my mind, is any kind of movement.

We all move, all the time. So just what sets dance apart from every other movement? Well, usually it's movement in response to music. Music and dance go together like any other well-matched couple. After all, even babies in the womb will "dance" when they hear music played. But you don't have to have external music to dance. The music can be in your head.

When you're dancing, you should also use all your senses. *Feel* every movement throughout your body, noticing where your body is in space at all times. *Smell* the honest odor of sweat as your muscles warm and work hard. *See* yourself in the mirror and notice the movement of the muscle under your skin as you work against gravity in your strength training exercises, or as you complete a complex movement. *Hear* the music, feel it thumping right to your very core, and notice how it drives your body's very motion.

This multisensory experience is part of the experience of dance, part of the art of fusing your mind and body together into one, and part of what makes the Rock Your Body workout unique.

Now, onto the specifics.

(continued)

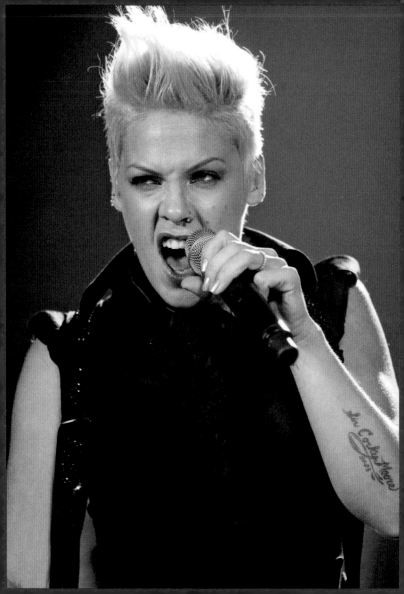

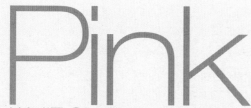

Pink

JAMIE ON PINK: I directed Pink's *Try This* world tour. She is an intense go-getter. Any challenge you give her, she's up for it. She can do everything, whether it's aerial work or hip-hop. You can see how she took her early gymnastic work and infused it into the world of entertainment and dance and created something fun from it. You can definitely tell she's an athlete. When I work with Pink, I always know it's going to be crazy and fun!

PINK ON JAMIE: Jamie is supercreative and diverse. He gets involved in every aspect of the tour, which is so much fun for both of us. He knows what the fu*k he's talking about. Some people are lucky or blessed enough to be able to change other people's lives with their talent. Jamie is one of those people.

Tony Selznick
On Rock Your Body

Tony Selznick, Jamie's longtime agent, wasn't surprised when Nike came along. "What sold Nike on Jamie was that he quickly showed them that they could go to him for everything, just like Madonna does: fashion, attitude, concepts on the billboards to commercials to live shows." Tony also knew that Jamie would be able to motivate people to actually do the workouts.

The same goes for the Rock Your Body workout, he says. "I've tried every dance video out there, and Rock Your Body is different because of the kind of director Jamie is and his approach to what he's doing," Tony says. "Jamie has his own inner rock star, and that's really important. It's the mind-set you have when you approach the move- ment that makes a difference. That's why Jamie is not just a great dance teacher but a great director and motivator. His approach makes you want to do it yourself after seeing the way he does it."

Learn to Breathe

Did you know dancers sometimes forget to breathe? I mean, they breathe enough to stay alive when they're performing, but too often it's shallow, quick breaths that do noth- ing for their form, energy, or strength, and too often I see them holding their breath.

So before you even start the workout, I want you to spend a few minutes breathing. Yup, that's right. In and out. But do it this way. Lie down on the floor and put one hand over your stomach. Breathe in through your nose to the count of three, deep into your diaphragm, until you feel your stomach rise. Then exhale slowly through your nose, also to the count of three, and feel your stomach deflate. Do this for about 2 minutes. This is also a great exercise when you're feeling stressed, overwhelmed, or anxious.

Now, when you start the workout, keep the Golden Rule of breathing in mind:

Breathe *out* on the part that requires effort. So, for instance, if you're doing a kick, breathe out as your leg kicks. But if you can't remember that, at least remember to breathe in and out deeply, without holding your breath!

Getting Started

So here's what I want you to do:

1. **Read through the next four chapters carefully.** Get comfortable with the moves and the pictures. Walk your way through each move five times before moving onto the next. As you go from one move to the next, try to visualize how the two moves fit together so that they become dance steps, not just individual exercises.

2. **Prepare your space.** You're going to need a fairly large, open space for this program. Your living room is fine; just push the couch and coffee table back against the wall. If you're dancing on the carpet, you can dance in bare feet. If you're on a hard floor, I want you in athletic shoes and socks.

The Rock Your Body Party

If you've watched the *Rock Your Body* DVD, then you can see how much fun all of us had learning the steps together. Face it, any kind of dance is more fun when you're doing it with other people. From the beginning of time, dance has been a communal activity. So I want you to throw yourself a Rock Your Body party. Invite two or three of your best friends—however many your space can manage—over to learn the routine and dance the dance. Promise them margaritas and chips and salsa afterward, or plan to go clubbing afterward for more dancing. Whatever— just make sure there's some fun reward at the end.

Give each of your friends a copy of my book (and no, this isn't just a way to sell more books!) and read through the movements together, practicing them one by one. Then pop in the music, stand facing front, and get ready to rock! Remember, you can also get a copy of the *Rock Your Body* DVD by visiting www.rockyourbodyprogram.com.

I don't have a set definition for success. I think success is personal. It's your own personal journey. So you have to define success for yourself . . . someone else's definition of success should not be yours.

3. **Dress for success.** If you've seen my *Rock Your Body* DVD, you've seen that my dancers wear every conceivable outfit for rehearsals. Baggy pants, cut-off T-shirts, leotards. Personally, I'm kind of a clothes hound. Even my agent calls me when he's ready to buy clothes. Here's the key advice, though: Wear whatever you feel comfortable in. My recommendation, however, is that you wear an outfit that doesn't hide your body. No matter how you feel about your body, the more you see it, the more you see it working, the more comfortable you'll become in it. So take a risk and put on those spandex pants and sports bra or clinging Pilates shirt. I want you to see how each movement looks on your body. Just make sure that whatever you wear gives you room for movement.

4. **Pick out your music.** The music is key. The most important thing is that it has an eight-beat. That means you can count to the tempo 1-2-3-4-5-6-7-8. Both routines are composed of smaller eight-beat routines, and all warmups and cooldowns are done to an eight-beat tempo. When you set the volume, whether it's on your MP3 player or your stereo, set it loud. I want you to feel the thumping within you.

Celebrities I've Worked With:
Ellen DeGeneres

I first worked with Ellen when I choreographed her opening number as the host of the Grammy Awards. Ellen is my favorite kind of dancer because her movement is infectious and comes from a place of pure joy. We love her. She makes us laugh. We want to dance with her! She's television's greatest dancing queen.

5. If you have the *Rock Your Body* DVD (available in stores and at www.rockyourbodyprogram. com), pop it into your player now. I want you to watch it all the way through at least once before you even start to move. Watch it with the book open in front of you and follow along with the DVD. Although you don't *have* to use the DVD during your Rock Your Body workout, it certainly won't hurt.

6. Drink half a bottle of water, or about 4 ounces of water. I want you hydrated *before* you start the workout.

7. Turn off the ringer on the land phone and on your cell phone.

8. Ignore the doorbell if it rings. FedEx can leave the package on your porch.

And what's the most important thing to do to get ready? Imagine yourself a rock star!

Let's go!

Celebrities I've Worked With: **Shakira**

Shakira has soul and spirit, especially when it comes to dance. And while she's not a trained dancer, her dancing is some of the most intriguing I've ever seen because it comes from her guts and soul.

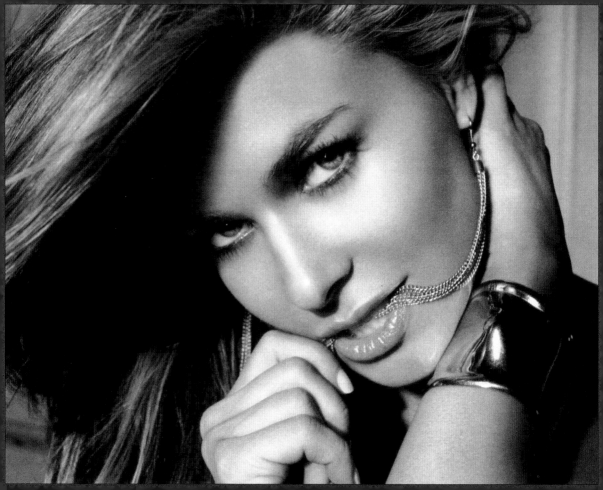

Carmen Electra

JAMIE ON CARMEN: Carmen Electra is an actress and dancer with an impressive body of work in the movies and television, on the stage, and with her own dance troupe, the burlesque cabaret act The Bombshells. An original member of The Pussycat Dolls, she and I have worked together for more than a decade.

CARMEN ON JAMIE: Jamie's choreography is bold, emotional, passionate, and explosive. He's a visionary who makes his visions come to life. Look what he's done with Madonna. No one else could have dreamed up such exciting concepts. He portrays women as very strong, and his choreography for us is as hard and powerful as it is for men. There's something incredibly sexy and empowering about that. Jamie's choreography also touches your body, heart, and soul. And his coaching stays with you. When he gives me something new, I go over it again and again until it's in my bones. No one gets things right away. But oh, when you do get his stuff, and you feel the energy he puts into every step and sequence, it's like flying.

Have **no doubts.** Anyone
——everyone—— **can dance!**

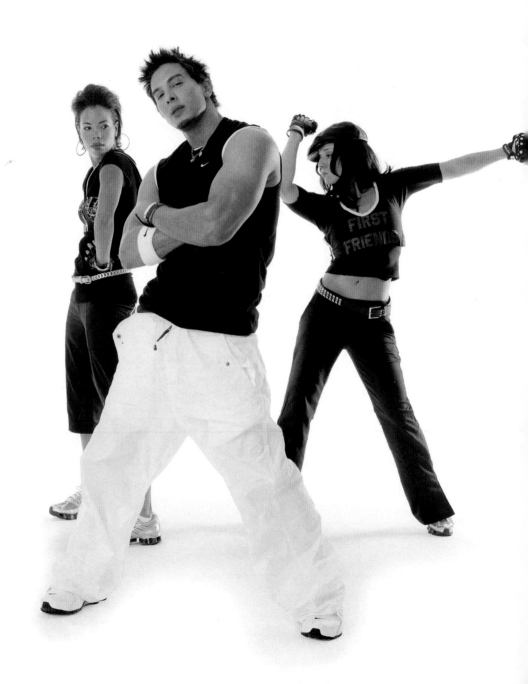

Chapter 5
Rock Your Body Warmup

I don't care how you arrange and rearrange the basic components of the Rock Your Body workout as long as you always include the warmup and the cooldown. Rock Your Body is a highly intensive workout, one that calls upon every part of your body. But if you've been sitting at a desk typing on a computer, or driving kids around, or even shopping, slamming right into any workout without warming up first would be like trying to go from zero to 75 mph in a car that's been sitting outside on a freezing night. You need to warm your engine.

The warmup I've designed here prepares you for the full routines by gradually increasing your heart rate and breathing so more oxygenated blood begins flowing throughout your body. An added bonus: This warmup is designed to not only get your muscles into the groove but your mind as well.

This is one of the few sections of the program where you can choose to do the individual movements as exercises or pull them together into one fluid dancing movement. It's up to you! And remember the advice from the previous chapter: Check with your doctor regarding any exercise routine before you start just to be sure you're good to go!

Okay, ready? Show me what you got!

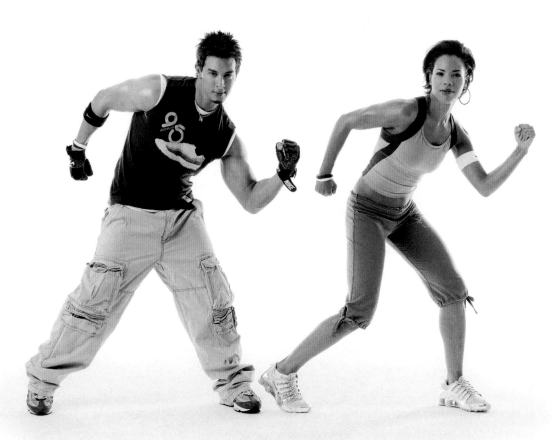

Catch Step

GOAL: Warm up and learn this "home base" position.

STARTING POSITION: Face forward with your legs slightly more than shoulder-width apart and knees slightly bent.

TIME TO MOVE: Curl your arms in front of your torso and, leaning slightly to the left, rock your torso twice to the left, then twice to the right, as you pump your arms up and down, keeping them bent at the elbow.

HOW MANY TIMES? Eight times (left *and* right is one set)

Return to this step between each of the following movements, maintaining your own movement to the music so the warmup routine becomes one fluid dance.

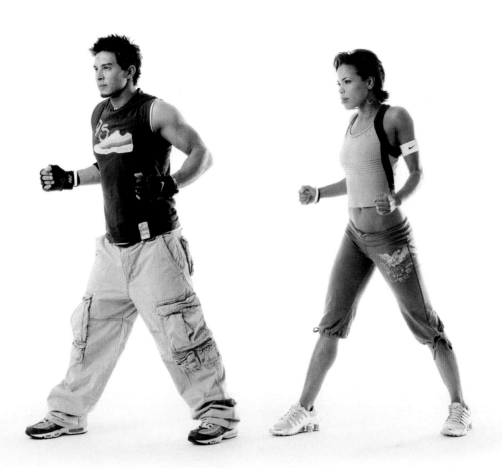

Shoulder Rolls

GOAL: Warm up the shoulder and neck area.

STARTING POSITION: Face front, legs slightly more than shoulder-width apart, knees slightly bent.

TIME TO MOVE: Slowly roll your shoulders forward, then up, then back in one smooth, circular motion in time to the music.

HOW MANY TIMES? 16 times

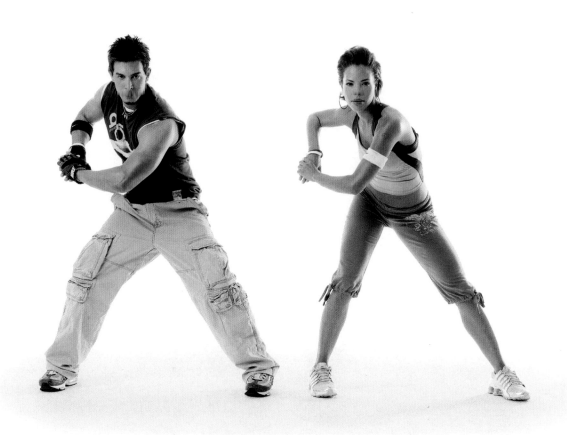

Groove Side-to-Side

GOAL: Warm up your torso and back.

STARTING POSITION: Face forward with your torso turned slightly toward the right on a diagonal and your legs slightly more than shoulder-width apart, knees slightly bent.

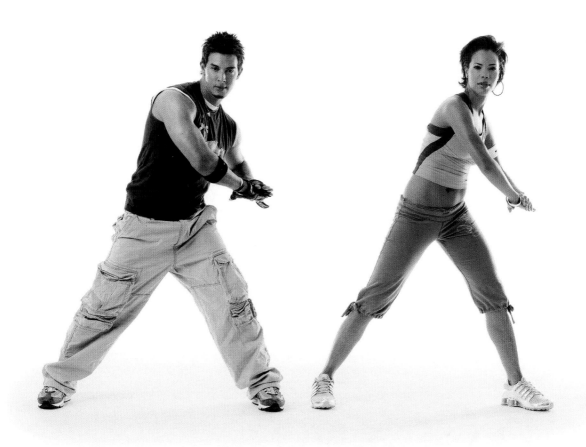

TIME TO MOVE: With your arms held chest high in front of you, elbows slightly bent, clasp your hands loosely and swing your arms and torso from side to side in a down and up rocking motion. Each side-to-side rock counts as one set.

HOW MANY TIMES? 16 sets

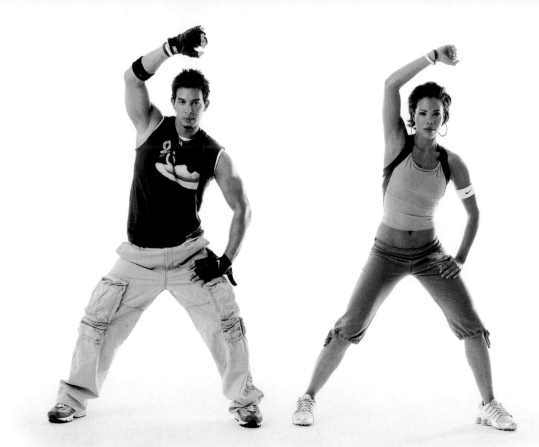

Hip Groove
and Arm Extensions

GOAL: Warm up your hips and arms in a full range of motion.

STARTING POSITION: Face front with your legs shoulder-width apart and a slight bend in your knees.

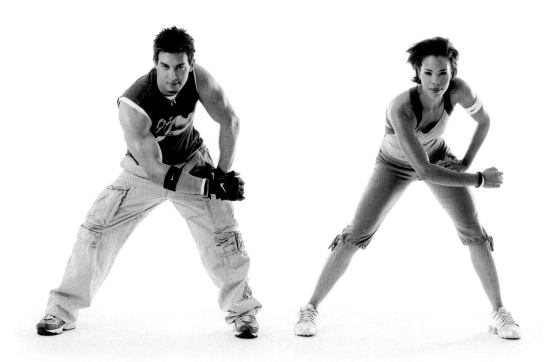

TIME TO MOVE: Rock your hips to the left then back as you swing your right arm above your head and down across your body. Complete 16 times to the left, then switch to rocking to the right, swinging your left arm up and down across your body 16 times.

HOW MANY TIMES? 16 times on each side

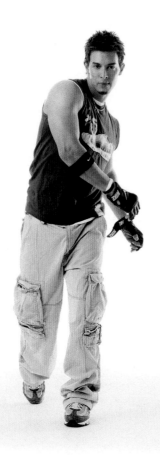
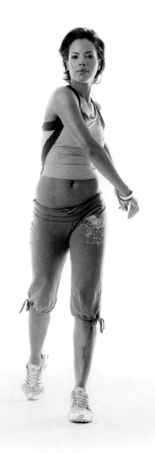

Walk and Shoulder Dips

GOAL: Begin moving your whole body while warming up your shoulders.

STARTING POSITION: Face forward, feet together.

TIME TO MOVE: Walk forward starting on the left foot. Left foot, right foot, left foot, right. Then tap your left foot forward while dipping your left shoulder down toward the right foot. Step together. Repeat on the right side.

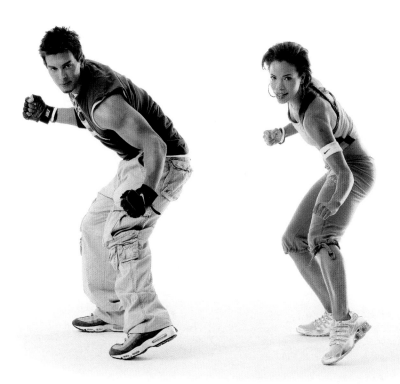

Now travel backward starting on your left foot for four counts, and repeat the left and right foot tapping and shoulder dipping.

HOW MANY TIMES? Complete the full movement forward and backward four times.

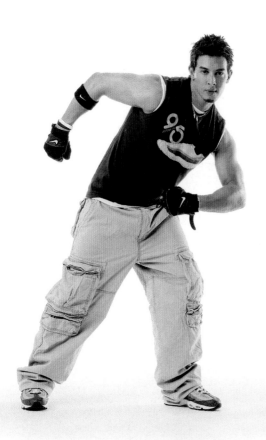
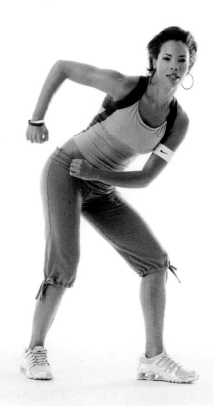

Soul Train

GOAL: Get the blood circulating in your legs and increase your heart rate so you're ready to dance!

STARTING POSITION: Face forward.

TIME TO MOVE: Keep your center of gravity low and your knees slightly bent as you step to the side with your left foot, then step behind with your right foot, then out again with your left in a "move-your-groove" grapevine, swinging your arms opposite the movement of your feet.

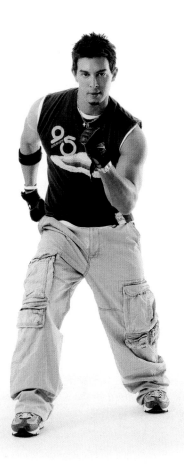
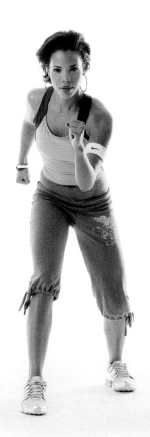

Now tap your right foot together with your left, but don't put your weight on your right foot because you'll be stepping out on that foot next .

Now step out on your right foot, then out with your left, then together. Right, left, together.

Repeat to the left.

HOW MANY TIMES? Perform the full sequence (grapevine, stepping out left and right) twice.

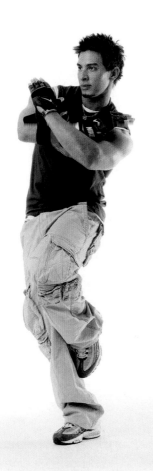
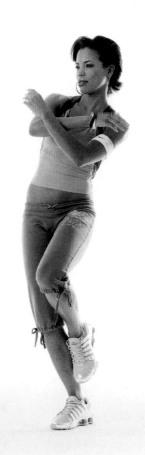

B-Boy Move

GOAL: Okay, now you're starting to get your groove on. Here's your first full-body, dance-based move. Let loose and let the magic flow!

STARTING POSITION: Face front.

TIME TO MOVE: Lift your left knee while crossing both arms in front of your chest, then extend your left leg forward on the diagonal to the floor and tap once while opening your arms

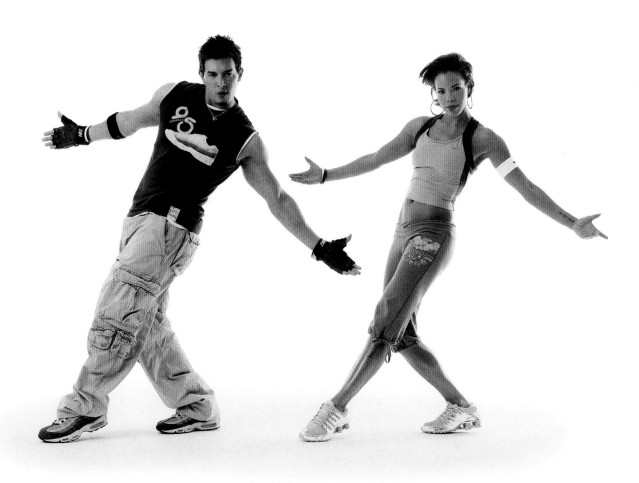

wide from their crossed position for a full range of motion. Now bring your left foot back to center, legs shoulder-width apart, crossing your arms in front of your chest, and repeat on your right side.

HOW MANY TIMES? Eight sets (left *and* right is one set)

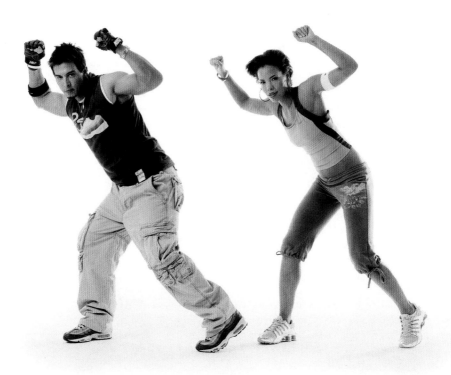

Rocking Pulldowns

GOAL: Continue warming up your arms, chest, and back.

STARTING POSITION: Face slightly right on the diagonal, arms held out at shoulder height, slightly bent at the elbow.

TIME TO MOVE: Rock your torso forward to the beat while raising your arms above your head then pulling them down two times to your shoulders (*see photo above*).

Continue the sequence by rocking your torso back as you cross your arms in front of your chest. Pull your arms in two times (*see top photo on opposite page*). Your arms should move in opposition to your body, so as your torso moves forward, pull your arms down to your shoulders; as your torso rocks backward, pull your arms into your chest. Complete the set (front and back) 16 times.

Maintaining the same rocking motion in your torso, drop your arms to your hips and swing your arms front and back in opposition to your torso movement (*see bottom photo on opposite page*). Complete 16 times.

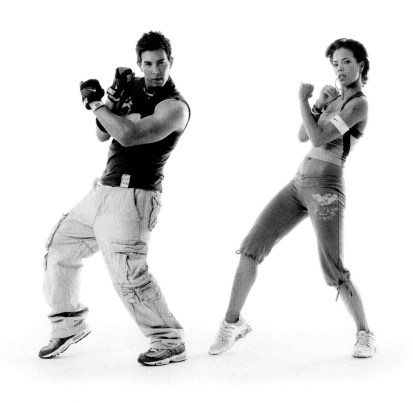

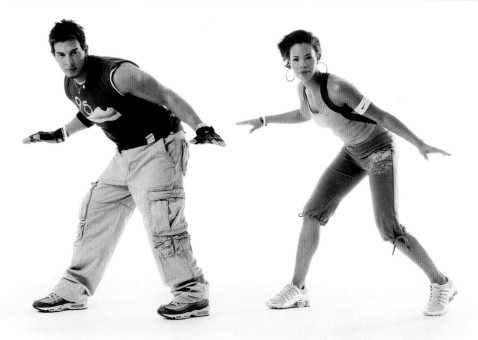

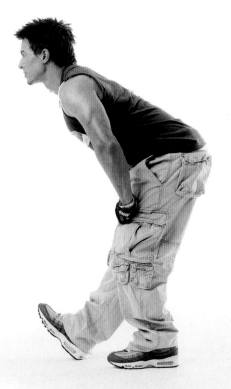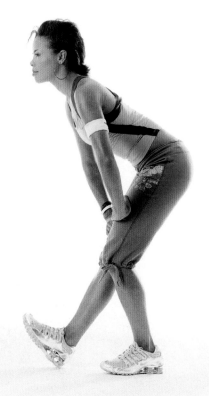

Hamstring
and Calf Stretch

GOAL: Elongate your muscles while you stretch out your hamstrings and calves, warming up your legs.

STARTING POSITION: Face right with your right leg extended and your foot flexed, hands on thighs.

TIME TO MOVE: Slowly let your chest drop while keeping your back straight and using your hands on your thighs to support you. You should feel a stretch in your hamstrings. Hold for a count of 32. Do not bounce!

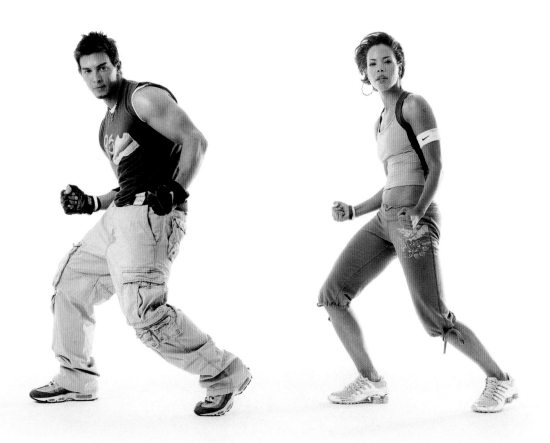

Now tap your right foot 16 times to the music to warm up your ankle, shin, and calf, hands still on your thighs.

Now incorporate your arms into the movement. Hold both arms in front of your body and pull them into your waist with every tap. Perform 16 times.

Repeat the entire sequence on the left side.

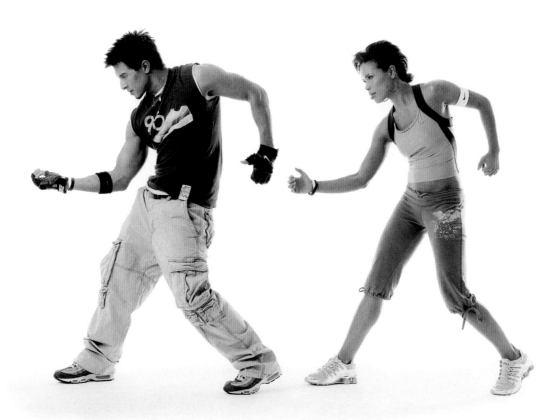

Guitar Move

GOAL: Warm up your entire torso and arms along with a little air guitar. Have fun with this movement; you're at your own concert rocking it out! One tip: Don't rush this movement, do it slow and steady.

STARTING POSITION: Stand diagonally facing right, feet apart.

TIME TO MOVE: Turn your left knee slightly inward while extending your right arm out and up as if you're holding a giant guitar. Swing your left arm down across your body in a giant

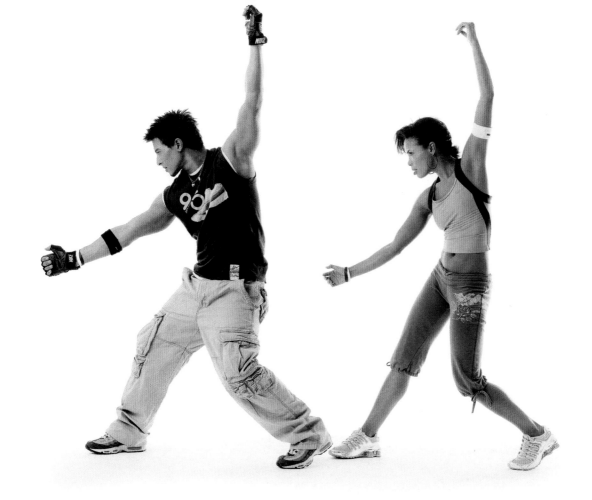

circular motion, then return your arm to the starting position. Your right arm never moves.

Repeat on the right side.

HOW MANY TIMES? Eight sets (one set is right *and* left)

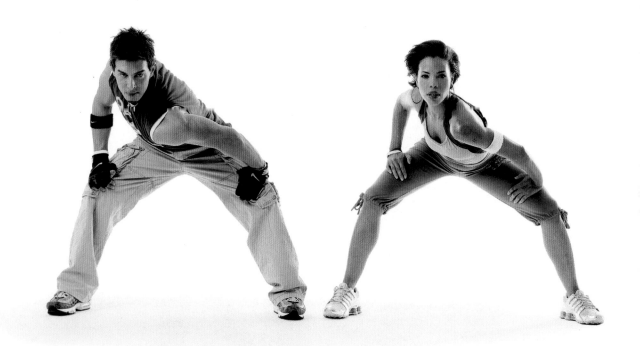

Torso Stretch

GOAL: To stretch your torso

STARTING POSITION: Face forward, legs slightly bent and feet shoulder-width apart, with your hands on your legs slightly above your knees.

TIME TO MOVE: Moving to the rhythm, lean your left shoulder down toward your right knee, then up, repeating the full down/up/down/up movement eight times. Now lean your right shoulder down toward your left knee, then up, again eight times. That's one full repetition.

HOW MANY TIMES? Eight to the right, eight to the left; four to the right, four to the left; two to the right, two to the left. Then slowly roll up.

Awesome!

You made it through the warmup.

Do you feel the blood pumping in your body?
Is your heart beating faster? Can you wipe a
thin film of sweat off your face?

Now you're ready to **Rock Your Body!**

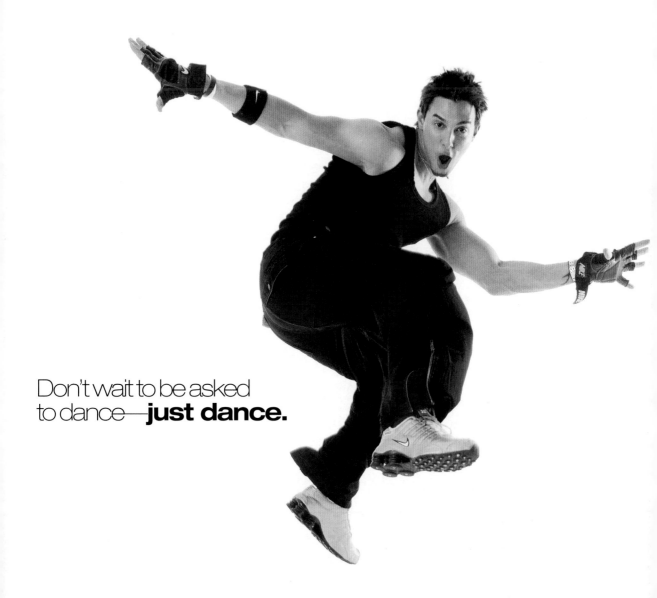

Don't wait to be asked
to dance—**just dance.**

Chapter 6
Rock Your Body
Strength Training

Y ou know you'll get an awesome cardio workout from the routines in the next chapter. But my Rock Your Body workout also provides you with strength training without the need for fancy machines or weights.

Strength training helps build your core. All this muscle building is one of the best ways to rev up your body's metabolism. The faster that metabolism roars, the more calories you'll burn in an hour—even if you're just lying on the couch. Combine the faster metabolism with the fat-burning routines in Chapter 7, and you're on your way to a much leaner, stronger body. You can do these exercises in the sequence I've provided, or you can choose to focus on the parts of your body you feel need the most work. Maybe one day you go through half the exercises, and the next day you go through the other half. But if you feel any pain, STOP! Rest that area for a couple of days before you return to the exercise for that muscle area.

Just keep a few things in mind: • Keep your chin up, shoulders down, neck stretched. No hunching! • Keep your stomach pulled in and your hips even. • Back straight—posture counts! • Focus on resistance to build up the muscle.

Start with the catch step from the warmup. Then move right into the first exercise.

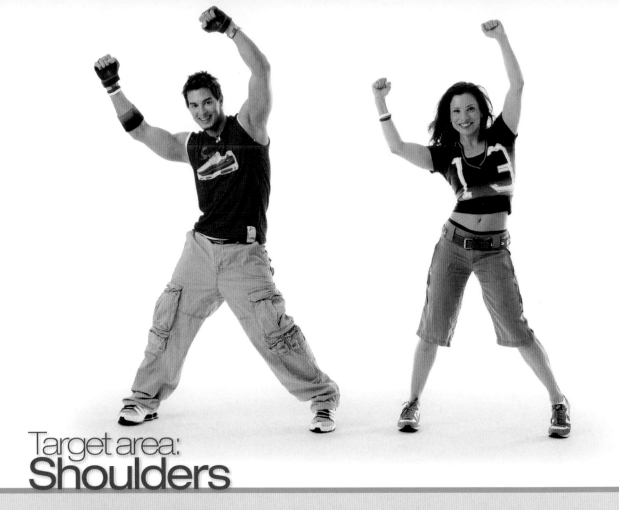

Target area:
Shoulders

STARTING POSITION: Face front, legs slightly more than shoulder-width apart and knees slightly bent.

TIME TO DANCE: With a little bounce in your step, rock your body to the left and push your arms out to the sides leading with your elbows. Now rock to the right and pump your arms overhead. That's one full set. Continue for a total of 16 sets.

Now step back with your left foot for one count, bounce for one count, then step together with your left foot for one count. Repeat on the other side.

Continue the total movement (left *and* right) for a total of eight sets, keeping your arms at shoulder height, pulsing upward leading with your elbows.

TRAINING TIP: Keep your elbows up throughout the entire set and never let them drop below shoulder height. You should feel a burning sensation in the muscles of your shoulders if you're doing the moves right.

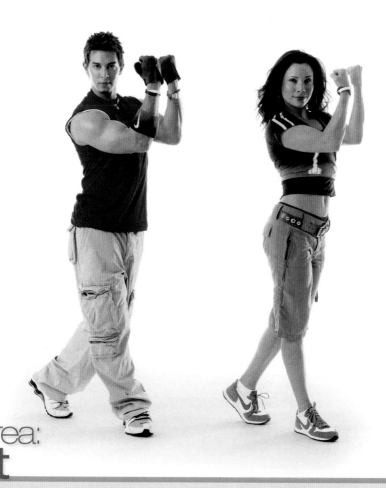

Target area:
Chest

STARTING POSITION: Feet together, arms by your side

TIME TO DANCE: Step forward with your right leg as you bring your elbows together in front of your chest with your hands closed into fists turned toward your face. Next, rock back to center, stepping your left leg in and opening your arms at chest level to prepare to repeat on the other side. Continue in a rocking motion for a total of 16 repetitions (right *and* left).

TRAINING TIP: Squeeze your chest muscle as you bring your arms together to increase the resistance.

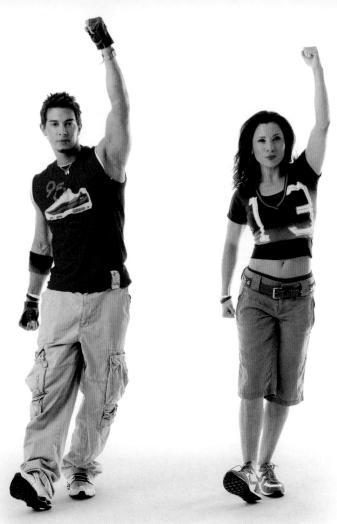

Target area:
Triceps

STARTING POSITION: Face forward, feet together, arms by your sides.

TIME TO DANCE: Step forward with your right heel while raising your left arm over your head, then bend your arm at the elbow to work the triceps and step together. Repeat as you step forward with the left heel, still working your left arm. Continue for 32 repetitions with the left arm, then 32 times with the right arm.

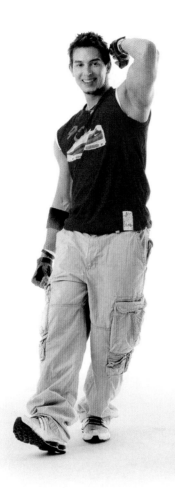
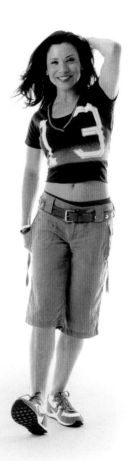

TRAINING TIP: This is not a quick, punching movement but a focused movement designed to provide as much resistance as possible. Also, your feet never stop moving throughout this entire movement.

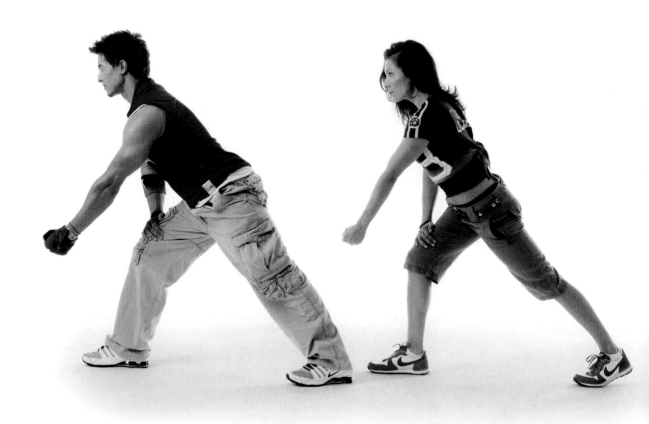

Target area:
Back muscles

STARTING POSITION: Face right on the diagonal, legs together.

TIME TO DANCE: Lunge forward with your right foot and your right hand on your right thigh, left arm extended forward. Slowly working against your own resistance, pull your left arm back toward your hip and maintain a straight plane with your back. Continue pulling your arm forward and backward a total of 32 times on the left, then switch sides and repeat 32 times, lunging your left foot forward and working the muscles in your right arm.

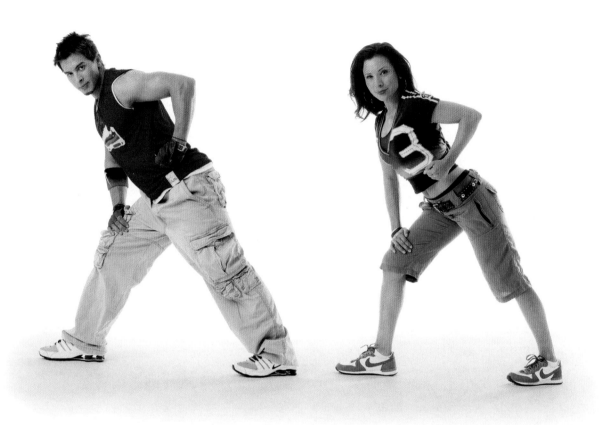

TRAINING TIP: You should feel a burning in your upper back and your rear deltoid muscle in your upper shoulder.

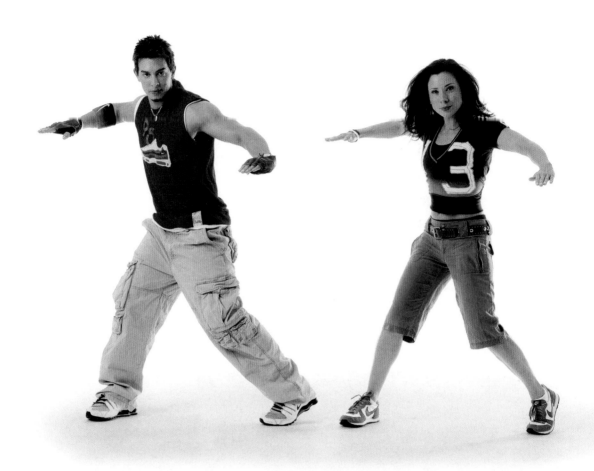

Target areas:
Chest and upper back

STARTING POSITION: Face forward, feet together.

TIME TO DANCE: Step out to the side with your left foot as you extend your arms straight out at shoulder height, open wide as if you were flying or opening a curtain. Bring your left leg center as you cross your arms together across your chest. Repeat with the right foot. Complete eight full sets (right *and* left is one set).

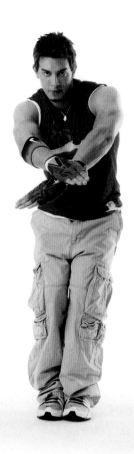
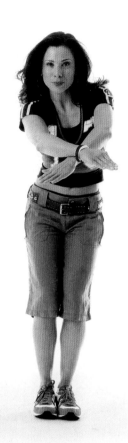

TRAINING TIP: Try to squeeze your shoulder blades together as you open and close your arms.

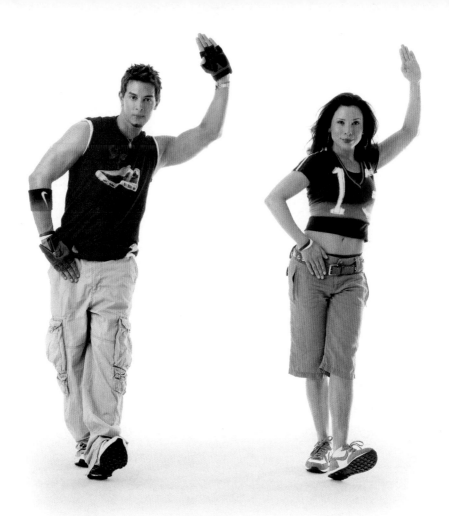

Target areas:
Legs, arms, back, and waist

(We call this our '80s Step because it looks like a retro move everyone used to do back then.)

STARTING POSITION: Face front, feet together.

TIME TO DANCE: Push your left heel forward, then together. Right heel forward, then together. Every time your heel goes forward, the arm on the same side swings up over your head; as the heel comes in, the arm swings down in a wide arc along your side. A full movement is left foot out, in, right foot out, in. Continue for 16 sets.

TRAINING TIP: You should feel resistance in your shoulder and back as you bring your arm around in a full range of motion.

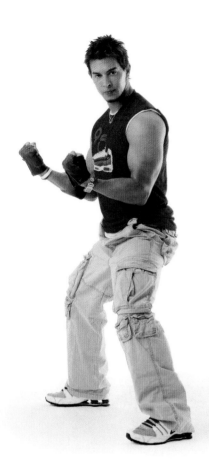
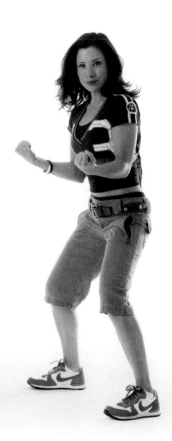

Target areas:
Legs and biceps

STARTING POSITION: Face right, feet together and arms by your sides.

TIME TO DANCE: Step your left foot out to the side, knees slightly bent as you curl your arms up to your chest, then step together and lower your arms. Repeat on the right side. Complete eight full sets (right *and* left is one set).

TRAINING TIP: Don't use your whole arm to create momentum when doing these curls because that prevents you from isolating your muscles. Instead, create resistance by keeping your elbows and chest raised and moving slowly. Also keep your elbows close to your sides. Make sure to squeeze your biceps every time.

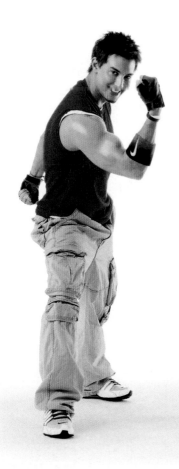
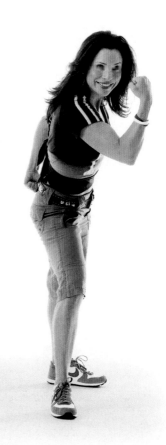

Target area:
Biceps

STARTING POSITION: Face front, feet together.

TIME TO DANCE: Step forward with your right foot as you curl your right arm up in a biceps curl and turn your body to the left. Return your right foot to center and face front. Repeat on the left side with the left arm. Complete eight sets (left *and* right is one set).

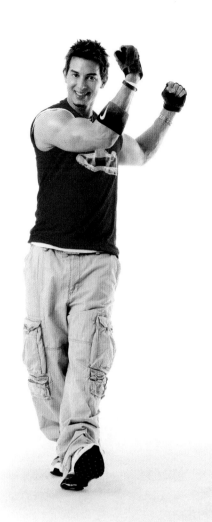
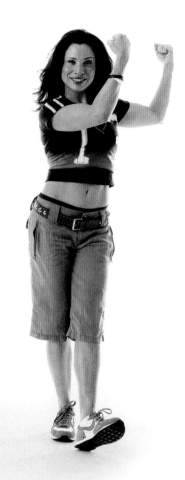

Target areas:
Abdominals and hamstrings

STARTING POSITION: Face forward, feet together.

TIME TO DANCE: Step forward with your left heel as you twist your torso toward the left, arms held at shoulder height, slightly bent. Twist, bounce, then bring your feet together, one movement to each count. Then step forward with your right heel and repeat. Complete 16 sets (left *and* right is one set).

TRAINING TIP: If you do the twisting movement correctly, you should really feel it throughout your obliques (the muscles along the side of your abdomen). Also engage your entire midsection throughout the move.

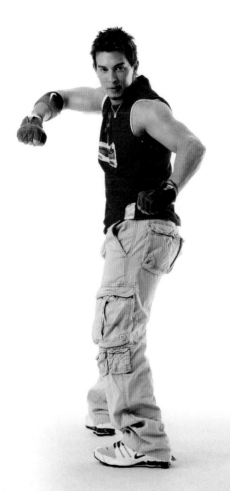
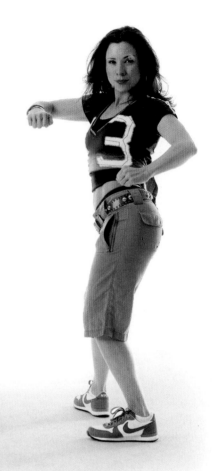

Target area:
Abdominals

STARTING POSITION: Face front, feet together.

TIME TO DANCE: Step forward on your left foot and then simultaneously twist both heels and your left hip forward as your upper body twists in opposition. Bring your body back to the front then step together. Repeat on the right side.

Complete eight sets (right *and* left is one set).

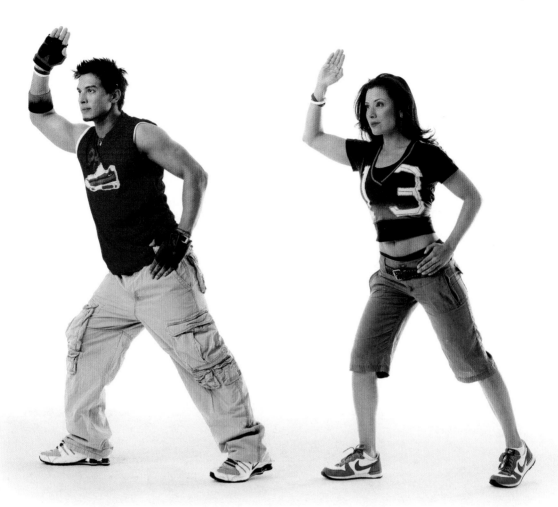

Target areas:
Abdominals, waist, and legs

STARTING POSITION: Stand diagonally facing right, left hand on your waist and right arm extended above your head, bent at the elbow.

TIME TO DANCE: Lift your left knee as you pull your right arm and shoulder down to the knee, crunching your torso, then return to starting position. Perform the move 16 times (up *and* down is one full movement), then repeat on the other side 16 times.

TRAINING TIP: Use a full range of motion so you feel the movement in your back, abs, and shoulder.

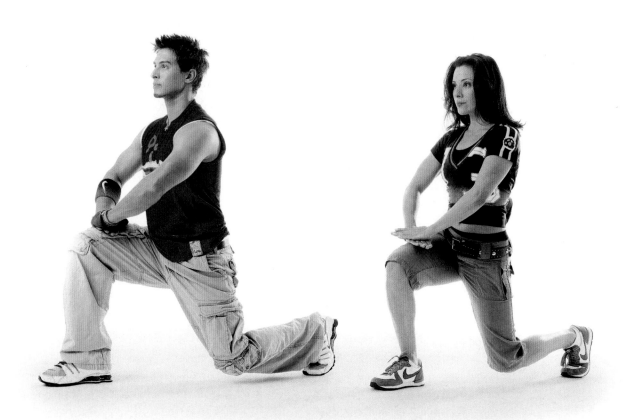

Target areas:
Hamstrings and quads

STARTING POSITION: Face right, legs apart.

TIME TO DANCE: Lunge forward on your right leg while keeping your left leg bent behind you. Keep your back straight as you lower yourself for four counts, release your arms, and pull them out to your sides as you rise up for four counts.

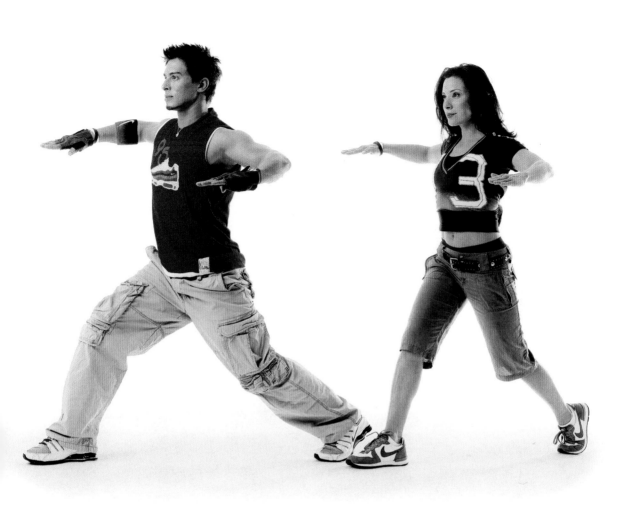

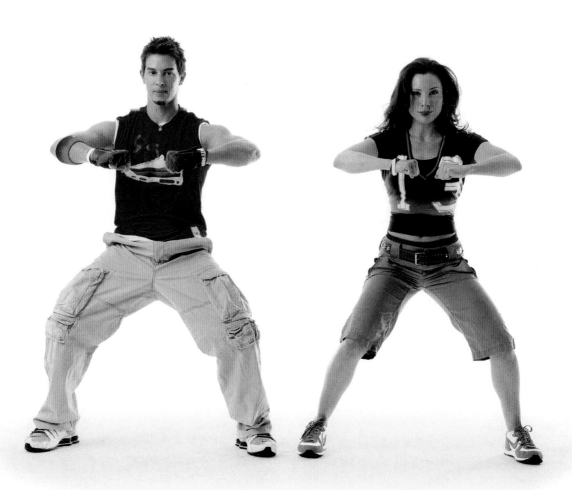

Target areas:
Legs and butt

STARTING POSITION: Face forward with your legs shoulder-width apart.

TIME TO DANCE: Bend your knees and drop your butt straight down, squeezing your butt tightly for four beats, then slowly rise for four beats. As you squat, keep your arms at shoulder height with your hands in fists in front of your chest. Complete eight sets (up *and* down is one set). Continue into the next move.

Now twist your torso in the opposite direction of your legs as you squat. This movement should feel more like a dance step as you squat, twist to the left, return to center, rise up. Squat, twist to the right, return to center, rise up.

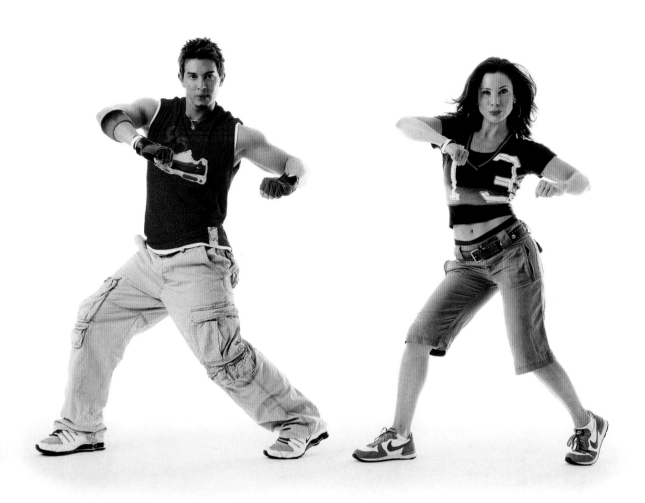

TRAINING TIP: Your butt should lead in the squat, almost as if you're sitting down in a chair. Keep your back straight and your knees over your toes.

You should feel a burn in the back of your legs and your upper thighs, or quads.

Whoa! Great job! Do you feel like Madonna or Usher when they dance? Well, you should! And I'll tell you what else you are—you're ready for the Rock Your Body routines! Come on!

Overcome fear and **self-doubt.** Be **confident.**

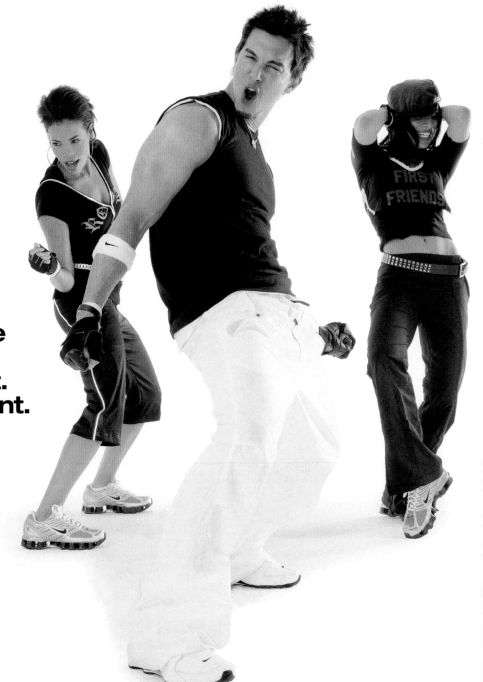

Chapter 7
Rock Your Body Routines

I have one question for you: Are you ready to dance? What? I can't hear you. Let me ask again: *Are you ready to dance?*

All right! Then you've come to the right chapter. Before you turn into the inner rock star you know that you are, let's get a bit of business out of the way. These dance steps are divided into eight counts. It's how dancers count the music and the steps. So a typical eight count goes 1-2-3-4-5-6-7-8. Each routine has five eight counts. It's that simple.

Still confused? Listen to the music before you start. Hear that underlying rhythm? Now count out eight beats. That's your eight count!

Sometimes, however, there's a beat in between the eight-count beats. So then the rhythm might go like this: 1-2-3-AND-4-AND-5-6-7-8. Generally, the extra beat means the movement is performed faster. In dancer lingo, this is called syncopated; all you have to know is that when you see the capitalized "AND", you've got an extra beat for the step, or an extra step in the routine.

Although the steps are broken up so we can match them to the pictures, the routine *is* a dance. I don't expect you to learn it on the first try, however. I want you to learn it the same way my dancers learn routines. Walk through the first eight count slowly. Then repeat it four times, each time getting faster.

Celebrities I've Worked With: Jennifer Lopez

With her curvy and sexy body, Jennifer Lopez is bringing sexy back. She's so dedicated and passionate about what she does that her passion is just contagious. I choreographed Jennifer on her hit music video "I'm Glad," which was an homage to the movie Flashdance. It was one of my favorite experiences because I was able to work with an unbelievably professional superstar and committed dancer, and we were able to re-create 1980s choreography—a great era for dance. Jennifer is no-nonsense. She has an amazing work ethic and is a trained dancer. She tries anything I ask her to do and never gives up. She's always on time and gives 100 percent more than she's asked to deliver. It's obvious why she's a superstar of music, film, and television. Most important, she's lovely to work with.

Now move on to the next eight count and again repeat it four times. Now put the first and second eight counts together and dance them seamlessly, with no break between, before moving on to the third eight count. After you learn the third eight count, put the first three together in one seamless dance, and continue on in this vein until you have the full routine down.

You'll spend at least an hour, maybe two, learning each routine. But once you have it down, the entire routine should take about 10 minutes. As you improve, you may find that you need faster music. By all means, shift your music. Find one with a slow tempo as you're learning, then one with a mid-range tempo when you feel more confident, and by the time you've got the routine down, go for it with something you can really rock to.

Another point: Not every step is depicted in a photograph, so don't worry if you don't see the step pictured.

Finally, there are two routines here. They're designed to be performed separately. After you finish the first one, take a 10-minute break, drink some water, catch your breath. Then go on to the second if you like, or save the second for another day and move right into the cooldown described in the next chapter.

Even if it seems too difficult,
push yourself—**keep going.**
That extra push will bring
real rewards.

First eight count

COUNT 1:

Slide your left leg forward, arms stretched above your head.

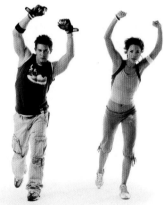

Count 1

COUNT 2:

Lift your right knee to your waist while simultaneously bending slightly toward your knee, arms at your sides . . .

AND: Step out on your right foot.

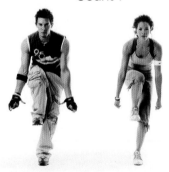

Count 2

COUNT 3:

Step out with your left foot . . .

AND: Now jump, bringing your legs together and crossing your right foot over your left while holding your arms straight out in front of you crossed at the wrists.

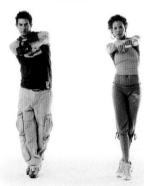

Count 3

COUNT 4:

Jump back, opening both arms and legs and landing with your knees slightly bent and your arms behind your legs.

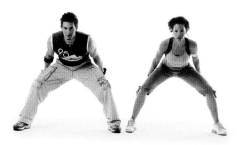

Count 4

COUNT 5:

Still in the squatting position, bring your knees in . . .

AND: Then out.

COUNT 6:

Then jump together, arms by your sides.

COUNT 7:

Slide back on your left leg while holding your arms as if you were running—right arm back and left arm forward.

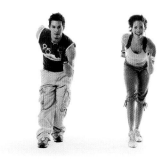

Count 7

COUNT 8:

Now step out with your right leg and raise your right arm, bent at the elbow, to your shoulder.

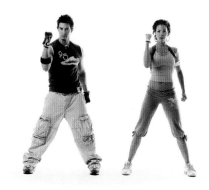

Count 8

Second eight count

COUNT 1:

Legs still apart, lean and lunge forward on your right leg with your body slightly twisted to the right as you grab your right wrist with your left hand.

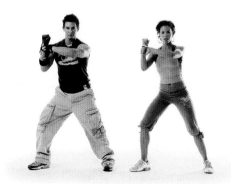

Count 1

COUNT 2:

Tap your left foot forward and across your right foot as you pull both arms to your hip and twist your torso to the left.

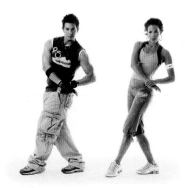

Count 2

COUNT 3:

Step your left foot back to center as you swing your arms (still holding your wrist) to the right . . .

AND: With your arms still connected, swing them down in front of your body to the left.

COUNT 4:

Then down and back to the right . . .

AND: Then down.

COUNT 5:

And back to the left.

COUNT 6:

After the swing to the left, release your hands and extend your arms in front of you.

COUNT 7:

Pull your arms, bent at the elbow, in toward your stomach as you slightly bend your left knee . . .

AND: Then extend your arms in front of you.

COUNT 8:

Turn and face front, hands by your sides, feet still shoulder-width apart.

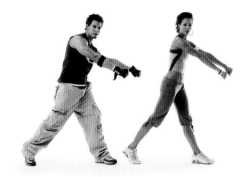

Count 6

Routine 1
Third
eight count

COUNT 1:

Still facing forward with your feet shoulder-width apart, step back with your left leg as you punch your left arm down across your body toward the floor.

COUNT 2:

Step out with your left foot, arms by your side.

COUNT 3:

Step behind with your right foot and punch your right arm down across your body toward the floor.

COUNT 4:

Step out with your right foot, arms by your side.

COUNT 5:

Now bring your right knee up while your left arm crosses your body at shoulder height, right hand raised to touch your left as if telling someone to stop. Squeeze your abs tight for balance.

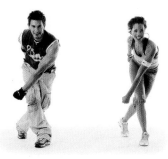

Count 1

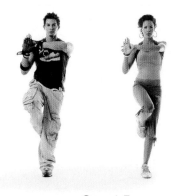

Count 5

COUNT 6:

With your hands still touching, swing them down to the inside of your right knee . . .

AND: Keeping your leg bent, push your knee around to the right and slowly lower it.

COUNT 7:

Straighten your right leg and step behind your left.

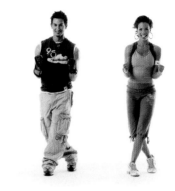

Count 7

COUNT 8:

Then step out with your left foot so your feet are shoulder-width apart as you roll your shoulders forward.

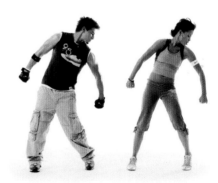

Count 8

Routine 1
Fourth eight count

COUNT 1:

Scuff your right foot along the ground and lift up at the knee.

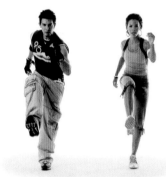

Count 1

COUNT 2:

Step out to the right . . .

AND: Step back with your left foot.

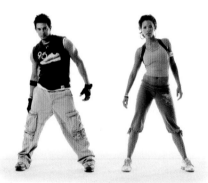

Count 2

COUNT 3:

Step forward with your right foot and punch your left arm down.

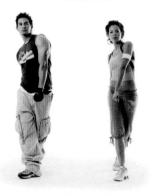

Count 3

COUNT 4:

Step together.

(Think of the jumping in and out of this next move as a jumping jack.)

COUNT 5:

Now jump your feet apart, knees bent and arms open at shoulder height . . .

AND: Then jump together, bringing your arms down by your sides.

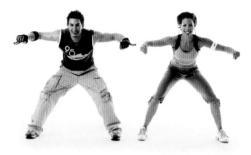

Count 5

COUNT 6:

Then lift your left knee up as your right arm crosses over your chest to the left as if you're marching . . .

AND: Step together.

COUNT 7:

Jump your feet out, knees bent and arms open at shoulder height (same as count 5)

AND: Jump together.

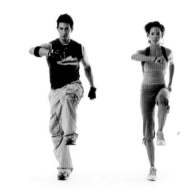

Count 6

COUNT 8:

Then lift your right knee up as your left arm crosses over your chest to the right as if you're marching.

Routine 1
Fifth
eight count

COUNT 1:

Step out with your right foot, your arms diagonally pushing away from your body as in the photograph.

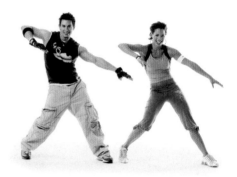

Count 1

COUNTS 2 and 3:

Push your chest out and rotate it to the back in a fluid counterclockwise motion, using your abdominal muscles to isolate your chest as it moves, arms held up at shoulder height to keep you balanced . . .

AND: Thrust your chest forward and your hips back while your arms, held at shoulder height and bent at the elbows, push back.

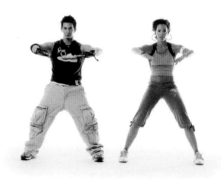

Count 3

COUNT 4:

Then push your chest back and your hips forward while your arms, still at shoulder height and bent at the elbow, push forward. Think of Shakira's amazing dance moves while doing this.

COUNT 5:

Cross your left arm over your right, then punch both arms down on the diagonal to the right as shown in the photo.

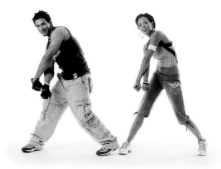

Count 5

COUNT 6:

Rock your body to the left and open your arms out to your sides in a low "v".

COUNT 7:

Then, with your right arm crossed over your left, punch both arms down on the diagonal to the right.

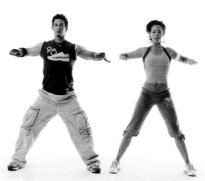

Count 6

COUNT 8:

Straighten and rock your body to the right, arms held thigh high and opened slightly.

Routine 2
First eight count

COUNT 1:

Step back with your left leg as you turn to face right. Leaning slightly forward, bounce your left leg behind you as your left arm, bent at the elbow, comes up chest high (as if you were walking).

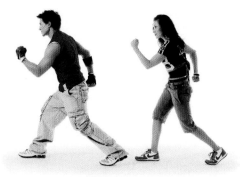

Count 1

COUNT 2:

Tap your left foot forward as you switch arms and, still keeping some bounce in the move, bring your right arm up.

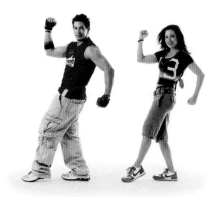

Count 2

COUNT 3:

Then with a little bounce, step your left foot back and, swing your arms back to the same position as in Count 1 (left bent, right back).

COUNT 4:

Twist to the left with your right arm in front, bent at the elbow in the running position.

COUNT 5:

Step back with your left leg as you pull your arms behind your back; clasp your hands together and lean forward.

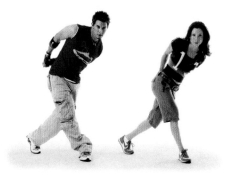

Count 5

COUNT 6:

Step out with the left foot and release your hands.

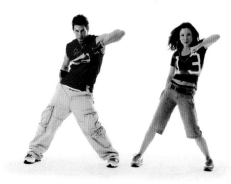

Count 7

COUNT 7:

Pump your left elbow up as in the picture.

COUNT 8:

Pump your left elbow up again.

Routine 2
Second eight count

COUNT 1:

Facing front, step forward on your left leg.

COUNT 2:

Extend your right arm in front of your body and push it toward the right as if opening a door . . .

AND: Then step back with your left foot so your feet are together.

COUNT 3:

Step your right foot forward.

COUNT 4:

Extend your left arm in front of your body and push it toward the left as if opening a door (same as in Count 2, but on the opposite side).

COUNT 5:

Now scoop your left arm to the left, holding your right arm slightly bent behind your back as in the photo.

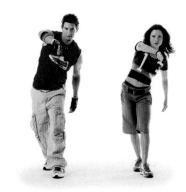

Count 2

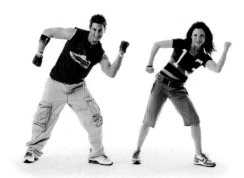

Count 5

COUNT 6:

Repeat the scoop with your right arm, leaning to the right.

COUNT 7:

Scoop your left arm to the left and step behind with your left foot . . .

AND: Step out with your right foot.

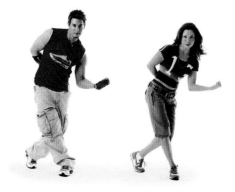

Count 7

COUNT 8:

Now step forward on your left leg, leaning forward with your right arm up and bent at the elbow and your left arm stretched straight behind your back.

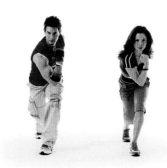

Count 8

Routine 2
Third eight count

We start out this routine with what we fondly call "the pimp walk." Give it some attitude. Remember . . . no one is watching! This is just a rehearsal.

COUNT 1:

Step forward on your right foot as you punch your left arm down across your body.

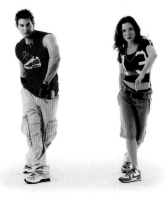

Count 1

COUNT 2:

Then slide your left foot slightly behind your right and pop your right toe up. Your body leans back with your weight on your left foot.

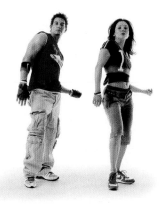

Count 2

COUNT 3:

Repeat Count 1.

COUNT 4:

Repeat Count 2.

(You will be traveling forward with these steps.)

COUNT 5:

Now hop back on your right foot simultaneously popping your left knee up along with your arms (as shown in the picture) . . .

AND: Put your left foot down.

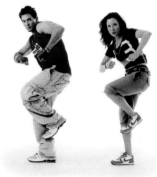

Count 5

COUNT 6:

Repeat Count 5 . . .

AND: Put your right foot down.

COUNT 7:

Repeat Count 5 . . .

AND: Put your left foot down.

COUNT 8:

Repeat Count 5.

(Since you're traveling backward with each hop, you should now be back where you started at the beginning of this eight count.)

Routine 2
Fourth eight count

COUNT 1:

Step out with your left foot and extend your left arm out to the side . . .

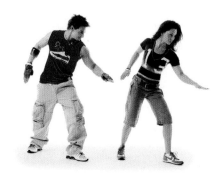

Count 1

AND: Step out with your right foot, arms waist high held out to the sides.

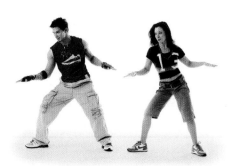

Count 1 "AND"

COUNT 2:

Punch your right arm down with your left arm held behind you.

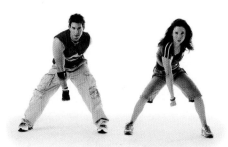

Count 2

COUNT 3:

Then jump your feet together while leaning back slightly, your right hip shoved forward and your right arm wrapped in front of your waist while your left arm wraps behind your back.

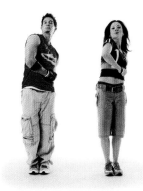

Count 3

COUNT 4:

Unwrap your arms and clap your hands up to the left by your head.

COUNT 5:

Now step out with your right foot, elbows shoulder height, and bounce right.

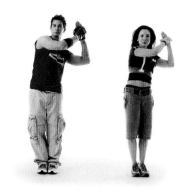

Count 4

COUNT 6:

Then bounce left, arms extended overhead.

COUNT 7:

Now bounce right again, elbows shoulder height.

COUNT 8:

Bounce right again, but lower, bending your knee and squatting.

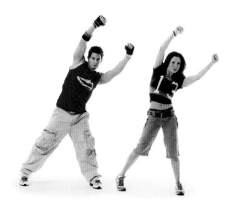

Count 6

Routine 2
Fifth
eight count

The first few counts of this move have you walking in a circle.

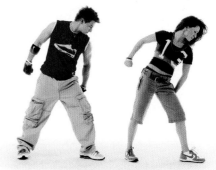

Count 1

COUNT 1:

Starting on your left foot, begin the circle walk to the left.

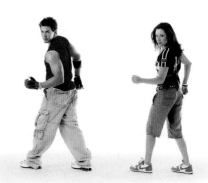

Count 2

COUNT 2:

Step right in the circle.

COUNT 3:

Step left in the circle . . .

AND: Bring your right knee in to your chest and your left elbow across your body to meet your knee.

COUNT 4:

Return to your starting position, stepping your right foot and bringing your elbow up above your head.

COUNT 5:

Slide your right leg forward diagonally right as you shoot your left arm across your body, your right arm stretched behind you.

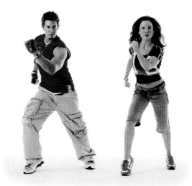

Count 5

COUNT 6:

Repeat the slide to the left, right arm shooting across your body, left arm stretched behind you.

COUNT 7:

Jump your feet apart with a slight bend in your knees as you punch both hands down between your legs.

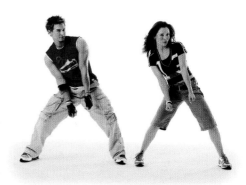

Count 7

COUNT 8:

Jump your legs together and hit your final pose.

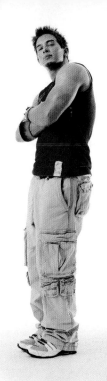
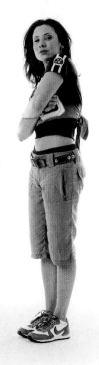

Final Poses

The final pose is just what it sounds like—the moment when you stop moving, face the audience, and wait for your thunderous applause. Give it some attitude! And feel good about yourself. You've just completed the Rock Your Body workout and have only the cooldown left.

While I have a final pose here for you to imitate, I really recommend that you experiment with your own. Listen to your inner groove and hidden rock star and make this move your own. You can see other options on the opposite page.

Face to the right with legs together, left shoulder lifted a bit higher than right and arms crossed in front of your chest.

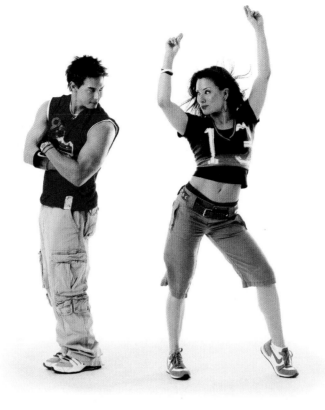

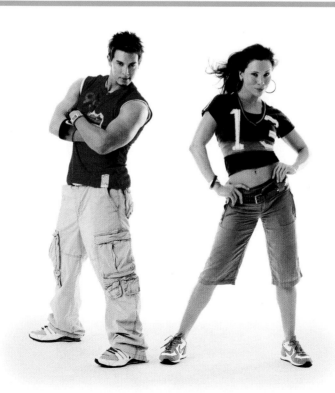

Create.
Love.
Be **happy.**

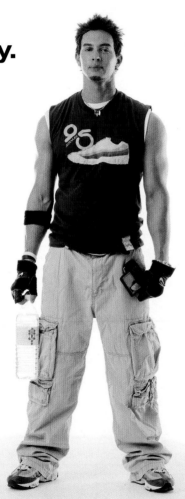
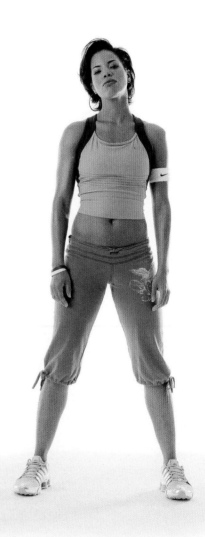

Chapter 8
Rock Your Body Cooldown

I am so unbelievably proud of you. You did an amazing job on the routines, and I hope you feel that inner glow all dancers get. But more important, I hope you're proud of yourself for what you just accomplished. You found your inner rock star, rocked your body, burned several hundred calories, strengthened and lengthened your muscles, and found a new outlet for expression. All that in just an hour or so!

Now it's time to cool down. Yeah, I know, you'd be quite happy to just hit the showers now. But if you do that, you're going to feel it tomorrow. This cooldown is designed to return your heart rate to normal and release any lactic acid buildup in your muscles that could cause soreness tomorrow. It's a wonderful way to reenter the "real" world while still maintaining all the benefits of your workout.

Important: Don't stop moving throughout this entire sequence. Keep swaying, rocking, or even stepping in place, but don't stop.

Ready? Nice and easy . . .

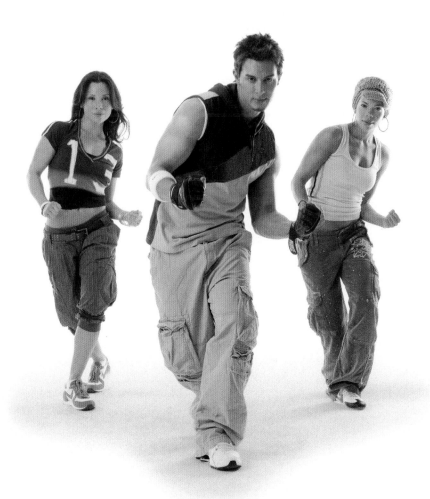

Walk Forward

Step forward with your left foot and bounce two times as you pull your arms to your waist.

Then step forward with your right foot (in front of your left foot), and bounce slightly two times as you pull your arms to your waist.

Walk forward with this move for eight counts: step left and bounce, step right and bounce, step left and bounce, step right and bounce.

(The next routine will return you to your starting place.)

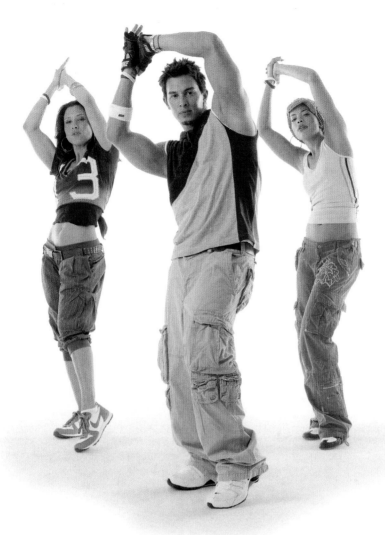

Overhead Clap

Now walk backward four steps (left, right, left, right) slightly on a diagonal, swinging your arms open as you step with your left foot and clapping above your head as you step with your right foot.

Complete four sets (forward *and* backward).

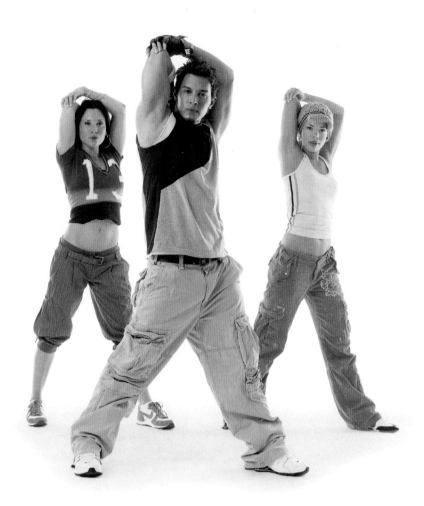

Arm Stretch

Now step out with your right foot, take a deep breath and swing both arms above your head, then slowly bend your left elbow and use your right arm to gently pull your left arm down for a good stretch. Hold the stretch for 16 beats.

Repeat on the left side, this time stretching your right arm.

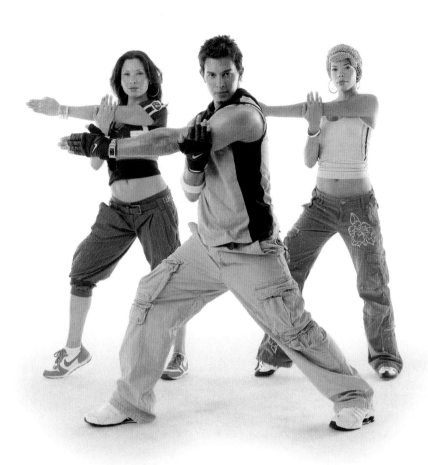

Arm Cross

Now release your arm from behind your head and use your right hand to pull your left arm by the elbow across your chest at shoulder height. Repeat on the other side. Hold each stretch for 16 beats.

Release and drop your arms and walk in a circle to the left for eight beats (left-right-left-right-left-right-left-right). At the end of the circle walk, tap your right foot together with your left and end up with your body facing to the left so you're ready to transition into the next step.

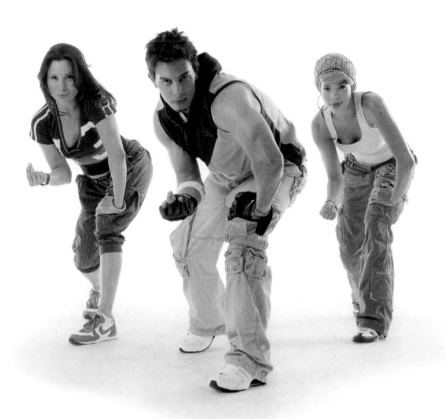

Step Touch

After you finish the circle walk, step your left foot forward and tap your right foot as you rock your body down, arms bent at your hips. Then step back on your right foot and tap your left foot, leaning your body back. Repeat the forward and backward tap in a type of electric slide.

Now walk the circle to the right, starting on your right foot. Right-left-right-left-right-left-right-left. Finish the circle walk by tapping your left foot together with your right and facing slightly to the left so you're ready to transition to the next step.

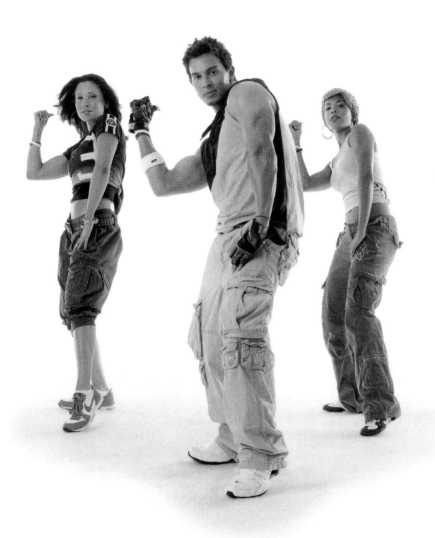

Now step forward on your left foot and tap your right, leaning your body forward, then step back on your right foot and tap with your left, leaning back. Repeat the forward and backward tap.

This entire sequence—the circle left, tapping front and back, then circle right, tapping front and back—is one set. Complete four sets.

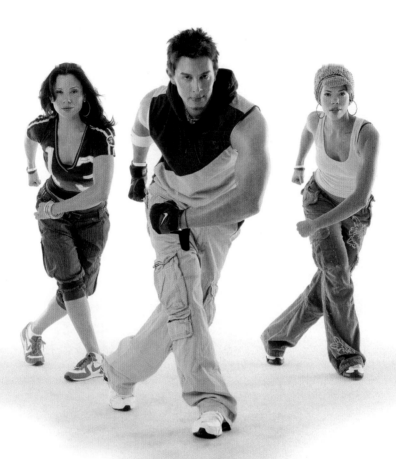

Cross Step

Now facing front, cross your right leg forward over your left, leaning forward with your left arm across your chest and your right arm behind you.

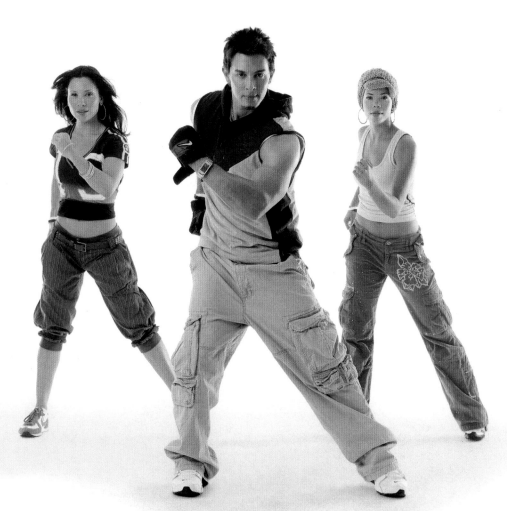

Cross Open

Then step out with your left foot, your left arm across your chest and right arm behind. Travel forward for 16 beats.

Starting with the right foot, march backward for eight beats.

Complete four sequences (the entire sequence begins with crossing your right foot over your left and ends with the backward march).

Finish facing forward and step together. Take a deep breath, drop one arm, leaving the other above your head, and take a bow.

You're a rock star!

Part III
Rock Your Diet

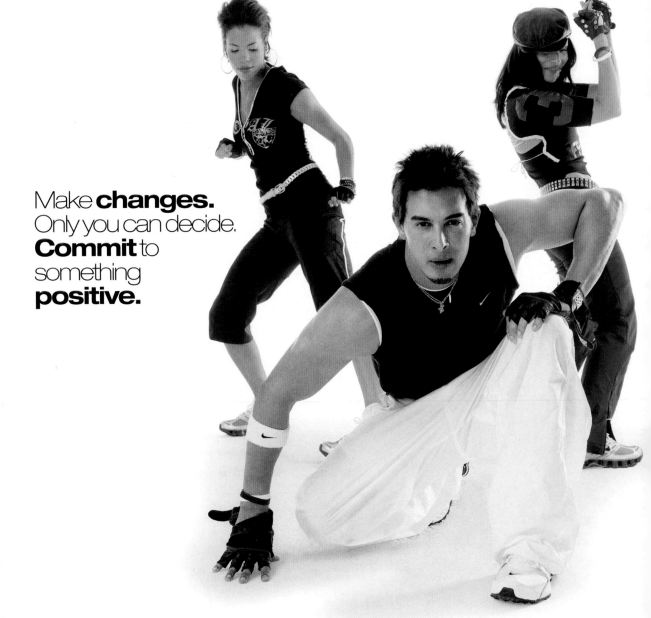

Make **changes.**
Only you can decide.
Commit to
something
positive.

Chapter 9
The Dancer's Diet

I f you've ever watched ballerinas dancing and marveled at the strength and power in those slim bodies, then you've seen the power of nutrition at its finest. Contrary to what you might think when you see a thin, willowy dancer, however, she isn't living on cigarettes and yogurt. In fact, the International Association for Dance Medicine and Science estimates that a 19-year-old dancer weighing 110 pounds needs at least 1,900 calories a day for peak performance.

Whether it's ballet, hip-hop, or ballroom dancing, I'm here to tell you that without eating right, no dancer is going to make it. Now, obviously, I'm not a nutritionist. But after more than 15 years of dancing and working with dancers, I think I've learned a thing or two about the right—and wrong—way for dancers to eat. Still, just to make sure I'm not sending you in the wrong direction, I've called in the expert, Debra Wein, MS, RD, of Sensible Nutrition in Boston, the nutrition consultant for the Boston Ballet. She also teaches at the Boston Ballet school and has been interviewed about nutrition by just about every major magazine you can find on newsstands.

She agrees with me: To fuel your dancing body, you need the right mix of nutrients—that means carbohydrates, protein, and fat. But she also told me something I didn't realize: Without the right kind of diet, you won't get the micronutrients so essential to repairing muscle, strengthening immunity, and protecting you against a variety of health-related problems. Sounds important, doesn't it? After all, if you don't feel well, you can't dance. And if you can't dance, you'll only feel worse.

Another thing she stressed: Forget about starvation diets. "A body deficient in calories can't perform at its best," she says. "So getting adequate fuel is the first rule to live by." And if you don't?

"The first thing your body will do is make sure it can carry out its normal function," she says. If you're adding a high-intensity, endurance workout like Rock Your Body on top of a low-calorie diet, and you don't have the stored body fuel (i.e., fat) to carry you through, you're going to be in trouble. What kind of trouble? Like not menstruating, she says. It's called the female athlete triad. The triad is a common problem in female gymnasts, dancers, and other athletes. It's composed of an eating disorder (anorexia or bulimia, most often), stopping of menstruation, and osteoporosis, in which your bones weaken. While eating disorders are much less common in men, those in certain sports—such as wrestling—are prone to them.

But let's be honest . . . a much greater problem these days is getting too many calories. After all, there's a reason that nearly 65 percent of Americans are either overweight or obese.

I'm sure many of you bought this book hoping it would help you lose weight. It will—the workout, that is. If you stick with it, perform it at least three times a week, and if you follow what's in this chapter. I call the advice in this chapter the Dancer's Diet. Even though it has the word "diet" in the name, however, it's not a weight-loss plan. Instead, it's a road map to a way of eating designed to improve every aspect of your health. Still, if you're rocking your body as I've outlined in the previous section, and eating as I'm about to tell you, then you should start seeing pounds peel off as muscles take over for fat.

One Step at a Time

Do you know how most of us eat, dancers or not? Really awfully.

For instance, only about four out of 10 of us eat an average of five or more servings of fruits and vegetables per day, and at least a third of us get 41 percent of our daily calories from nutritionally empty foods high in calories.

And dancers? Well, the ones I see seem to live on junk food. Sodas, chips, doughnuts, fancy coffee drinks. It just amazes me.

Now, I'm not sitting here holding myself up as the god of nutrition. I don't believe in classifying things into "good" and "bad" and, as you learned in Chapter 1, I'm a big believer in balance. So sure, I'll hit the food court for a four-cheese pizza when I'm traveling. But not every day. Generally, I try to eat the way I recommend you eat—healthy proteins and fats; small, frequent meals; lots of salads and other vegetables and fruits.

I've been eating this way for nearly 15 years now, so it's become second nature for me to bypass the McDonald's at the airport and head over to the sushi counter. But it might take some getting used to for you. So I want you to take it slowly.

Start with changing one or two things every 2 weeks. For instance, maybe the first week you switch from regular soda to diet soda and from fancy coffee drinks to plain coffee. Work on that for 2 weeks. Why 2 weeks? Studies find that's how long it takes for something to become a habit.

After 2 weeks, add one more change—maybe switching all your dairy products to skim and low-fat. Continue on from there until you've made all the changes Debra and I recommend here, and you're living the Dancer's Diet.

Jamie's Mantra
On Eating

I think the most important thing when it comes to good nutrition and eating is to listen to your body. Your body tells you what's good for you. I mean, that piece of chocolate cake might look good, but after you eat it, how do you feel? Weighed down? Maybe that means you've been eating too many sweets lately.

Have you ever gone without eating fast food for about a month and then had a burger and fries? You get this greasy, bloated feeling from all the salt and fat your body is no longer used to. So my message here: Listen to what your body is trying to tell you. If you feel gross after eating something, stop eating it!

Having said that, remember one of my earlier mantras: Life is about balance. Don't cut out every form of rich, fattening food. After all, one of my all-time favorite foods is a cupcake from this incredible bakery called Sprinkles in Beverly Hills. Heck, if they're good enough for Oprah, they're definitely good enough for me!

Getting the Basics

As you saw in the Rock Your Body workout, I didn't try to get you doing entire routines or even entire movements all at once. Instead, I broke everything into step-by-step instructions. And I'm going to do the same with your diet.

Instead of simply listing meal plans, I'm giving you the basic instructions to build your own meal plan. If you understand the basic underpinnings of the Dancer's Diet, then together with the recipes provided in Chapter 10 you should have no trouble creating an unlimited number of daily and weekly meal plans. It's the dancer's version of the "give a man a fish" vs. "teach a man to fish" parable.

The three main steps of the Dancer's Diet—think of them as the plié, second position, and third position of the diet—have to do with the three macronutrients in food: carbohydrates, protein, and fats. Unlike many "diet" plans that fill their pages with percentages and numbers, I promise I won't do that. There will be no weighing or measuring of food, no tracking of calories or fat grams.

Instead (with apologies to the 10 Commandments), I provide my Top 10 Choreographer's Commands—broad guidelines that show you *how* to eat to supply enough fuel for the Rock Your Body workout and your own hectic lifestyle so you receive maximum benefits without maximum calories.

Choreographer's Command # 1: Know Your Carbs

Pity the carbohydrate. Like a rock star in rehab, carbs have gotten a bad rap in the past few years. After all, given the plethora of high-protein, low-carb diets that have been touted in recent years, it's no wonder so many people worry that if they let a forkful of pasta or a crust of focaccia past their lips, they'll blow up like a bad movie. Well, I'm here to tell you that all those people gorging themselves on bacon and eggs and passing up pasta, bagels, fruits, and vegetables are not dancing for me! If they were, they'd never make it past the warmup!

That's because carbohydrates provide the fuel for your muscles and workout. No matter what kind of carb you're eating—simple, complex, white, brown, fruit, candy bar—they're all broken down into simple sugars, or glucose, and then stored in your muscles and other parts of your body for use as needed. That stored glucose is called glycogen, and if you find yourself getting tired during the Rock Your Body workout, it could be because you don't have enough stored glycogen.

You know that dizzy, headachy feeling you get when you're hungry? You laughingly chalk it up to low blood sugar, but that's exactly what's causing it. The low glucose level in your blood means your brain is literally starving for fuel because your brain, unlike muscle, can't store glucose. It's like a computer without a hard drive—you have to continuously feed it information, uh, sugar. In fact, your brain soaks up about 800 calories a day in the form of glucose. So if you're having trouble remembering the Rock Your Body steps, ask yourself: "When is the last time I fed my brain?"

These low-carb diets often sold themselves by selling the idea that if you starved your body of glucose from carbohydrates, it would turn to stored fat for fuel. I got news for you . . . that's not where your body heads first. If your body doesn't get enough fuel from carbs and stored glycogen, it first turns to muscle for its supply, starting with skeletal muscle and then moving on to the liver. You can only imagine what that does for your stamina!

So while a low-carb, high-protein diet will show quick results, the results are not from fat loss but from the loss of water and muscle. And here's another reason why that approach is counterintuitive; surely you've heard it said that muscle burns more calories than fat? Well, that's not quite the way it works. What's really going on is that muscle cells are more active than fat cells (which are really nothing more than, well,

Rockin' Reality

A calorie is actually the amount of heat required to raise 1 gram of water 1 degree Celsius; if you're talking about the "calories" in that fast food burger, you're talking about kilocalories, or the amount of energy contained in that burger. That energy can either be used as fuel (burned by the "heat" of your body, aka your metabolism) or stored. Stored kilocalories, of course, are also known as . . . fat.

your body's version of a couch potato). That means the more muscle cells you have, the greater their need for energy and the more energy you burn. Or, put another way, the higher your metabolic rate.

Okay, getting back to carbohydrates. All carbohydrates break down into the same sugar in your body, whether the carbs come from a spinach salad or a piece of chocolate cheesecake. Why, then, do we talk about "simple" and "complex" carbohydrates?

Well, think about how you start a fire. You don't toss down a big piece of wood and then try to light it. You start with balled-up newspaper and twigs. Think of these as simple carbohydrates. Just as newspapers light immediately and quickly burn fast and hot, simple carbs break down into glucose within minutes, sending a huge amount of sugar into your bloodstream for a quick shot of energy. The problem? Just as fire consumes the energy provided by the newspaper in minutes, your body consumes the energy provided by those simple carbs very quickly. Once that sugar burns up, you'll find yourself hungry again.

But if you build a nutritional program like you build a fire, adding fuel that burns more slowly, you'll find yourself in a much better position. That's where "complex" carbs come in. These foods, things like beans and legumes, whole grains, vegetables, and many fruits, take longer to break down in your stomach thanks in part to their high fiber content.

Hidden Benefits

In addition to providing you with long-term fuel, the high fiber of complex carbs comes with extra health benefits, like reducing your risk of several cancers, including pancreatic, colon, and breast; slashing your risk of diabetes; lowering cholesterol levels; and, the one you might be most interested in, cutting calories. One analysis of several studies found that adding just 14 extra grams of fiber—about the amount in a bowl of high-fiber cereal—could lead to a 10 percent drop in the amount of calories consumed. What's this mean? Well, if you're eating 2,500 calories a day, a 10 percent drop saves you 91,250 calories a year—a possible loss of 25 pounds!

The Whole Truth

When you're looking for whole-grain products, don't be fooled by color alone.
Read the labels: the word "whole", as in whole grain, whole wheat,
whole oat, should be first on the ingredient list.

Fiber, for the record, can't be broken down by your body. So it's like free calories that fill you up without filling you out. Plus, it acts like a trap, slowing the rate at which sugar enters your bloodstream. Instead of a quick hit of energy, you get a slow, steady supply of glucose that, among other things, keeps hunger at bay. We call these foods low glycemic foods because of the slower, gentler rise in blood sugar they bring. Which means those "simple" carbs are . . . yup, high-glycemic foods.

So let's review: quick-flaming simple carbs or slow-burning complex carbs? It's a no-brainer, right?

So how do you tell if a carb is simple or complex? Ask yourself these questions:

1. **Is it white or brown?** "White foods," like white bread, regular pasta, white rice, regular bagels, etc., are carbohydrates with the "complexity" stripped out of them. Instead of white foods, choose brown: brown rice, whole-grain pasta, whole-grain bread.

2. **Is it processed or natural?** The closer a food is to its natural state (i.e., an apple vs. potato chips), the more likely it is to still contain the fiber and other nutrients that contribute to its complex nature. An added bonus: Sticking with "real" foods dramatically reduces the amount of salt and extra sugar in your diet.

3. **Are the words *sucrose, glucose, corn syrup,* or *sugar* among the first three ingredients?** If so, it's loaded with extra sugar and thus a simple carb.

4. **What does the label say?** Look for foods with at least 3 to 5 grams or more of fiber per serving.

So what does this carbohydrate stuff look like on the Dancer's Diet?

Instead of . . .	You choose . . .
A bottle of apple juice to slake your thirst and provide energy	An apple with a bottle of water
A bag of chips from the vending machine	A bag of peanuts
A plain bagel with butter	An everything bagel (preferably whole wheat) topped with hummus
Regular pasta with tomato sauce	Whole-grain pasta topped with ratatouille

Now you're rockin'!

Choreographer's Command #2: Pick the Right Fats

No way am I going to jump on the low-fat bandwagon. Every dancer, heck, every person, needs fat. It helps you feel full, is vital to repairing injury to muscles, forms the building blocks for important hormones (like your sex hormones!), and is an important fuel to get you through a Rock Your Body workout—or any other endurance workout, for that matter. Once you hit the 20-minute mark in an exercise routine, your body switches from carbs to fat to fuel your workout.

So how much fat do you need? Not my thing, guys. As promised, I'm not going to have you counting grams. I am, however, going to give you the four basic steps you need to get the right fats in the right amounts—with no effort at all.

Step 1: Skip the saturated. Saturated fat is the type that's solid at room temperature. It's the white streaks on the steak, the thick, greasy stuff left in the pan after frying hamburgers, and the butter you just slathered on your toast. It's the primary fat in animal and dairy products.

It's also the type of fat that clogs your arteries, raises your cholesterol, and contributes to heart disease. You want to treat your heart badly? Keep eating that saturated stuff. You want to improve your health? Cut down on it.

I say "down" vs. "out" because it's impossible to avoid saturated fat entirely—even foods high in "healthy" fats like those described below contain a small amount of saturated fat. I'm just asking you to be aware of the main sources of saturated fat and get it sparingly. What's that look like on the Dancer's Diet?

Instead of . . .	You choose . . .
Hamburgers	Turkey burgers
Buttered toast	Whole-grain toast spread with jam
Buttered vegetables	Steamed veggies sprinkled with fresh herbs and a squirt of lemon juice
A sirloin steak	Duck breast, without the skin
Cheese and crackers for a snack	A low-fat or fat-free container of yogurt
Ice cream	Gelato or a frozen fruit bar

Step 2: Fall in love with olive oil. It's as close to an ideal fat as a fat can be. Olive oil is primarily a monounsaturated fat, which studies find helps lower bad cholesterol and raise good cholesterol—a recipe for a healthier heart if ever there was one. The beauty of olive oil is that it's like wine—there are so many different types and flavors. Fruity and sweet and sharp and subtle. Whenever I travel, I try to pick up some olive oil, particularly if I'm in a wine-producing region. So experiment!

As for what to do with it . . . well, how about the following:

- Pouring a puddle on your bread plate, sprinkling it with sea salt, and using it instead of butter for your bread.
- Using it to sauté every kind of vegetable, meat, poultry, or seafood imaginable. Oh, by the way, it's a myth that olive oil can't be used for high-heat cooking. I eat in some of the finest restaurants in the world, and olive oil forms the basis for nearly every dish.
- Mixing it with one-third balsamic vinegar and adding a pinch of salt and pepper plus a crushed garlic clove and calling it salad dressing. Much better for you than most bottled dressings, which are full of saturated fat, sugar, and preservatives.

Step 3: Seek out essential fatty acids. Bet you didn't know that fish are fatty. Well, they are, especially fish like tuna and salmon. And the fat in this fish is like liquid gold to dancers. It's called omega-3 fatty acid, and not only is it critical for good health and brain power (your body can't produce it on its own), but also lots of studies find it can reduce inflammation.

Inflammation is why your muscles ache after an intense workout. It's what contributes to heart disease. It's actually behind nearly every chronic disease out there, from diabetes to Alzheimer's to arthritis. But essential fatty acids like omega-3 fatty acids act like the oil in your car engine, preventing friction by quelling inflammatory chemicals and cells and keeping them from getting out of control.

Ideally, you should get two servings of a fatty fish each week. And don't forget fishy foods like tuna salad, salmon croquettes, and smoked salmon—they all count!

But what if you don't like fish? Here are a few other ways to get your essential fatty acids:

- Sprinkle flaxseeds over your yogurt, mix it into your cereal, or stir it into your morning energy drink. Flaxseeds are the vegetable world's equivalent of salmon when it comes to omega-3 fatty acids.
- Take fish oil supplements every day.
- Use walnut oil (another good source of omega-3s) for cooking and salad dressing .
- Get at least one healthy serving of greens every day—mustard greens, beet greens, kale, collards, spinach.

Step 4: Take out the trans. By now, you've undoubtedly heard about trans fats, the bad boy of the fat continuum. These man-made fats, which help make processed foods shelf stable and are used to fry most commercial foods, are to your heart what an empty arena is to a rock star—death. Heck, even New York City has banned them! Luckily, it's become much easier to know if you're eating trans fats since they now have to be listed on food labels, which has prompted many food manufacturers to drop them altogether. Follow their lead—make your diet trans-fat free.

Choreographer's Command #3:
Power Up the Protein

And now we come to the third major component of the Dancer's Diet: protein. You need protein to build strong muscles and strong bones, and to keep your ligaments and tendons (the soft stretchy parts of your joints) working right. Protein helps maintain the right balance of water, contributes to the manufacture of hormones, and keeps your immune system strong. If you're taking in more than you need, it can be burned for energy or converted into glucose if you need the extra energy; but if you don't need it, it gets converted to fat.

You don't need a lot of protein, however. In fact, it turns out most dancers (like most Americans) get way too much. Having said that, even the nutritionists don't agree on how much protein to get. The middle-of-the-road recommendation, though, seems to be about 0.6 to 0.8 grams per pound of body weight *for athletes*. If you're not an athlete (and most of you aren't), you need about half that. So, for instance, if you weigh 145 pounds, that's about 50 grams a day.

Now, I know I promised you I wouldn't make you count grams and I'm not going to, but just consider this: One chicken breast contains about a third of your daily protein needs. Add a cup of tuna and you're more than halfway there. Wash it down with a cup of skim milk and you've just hit your daily limit.

Why worry about the amount you're getting? I didn't know the answer to that question either, so I asked Debra. She told me that after your body has used all the important parts of protein (primarily amino acids), it has a bunch of nitrogen left over. That nitrogen combines with hydrogen, creating ammonia. The liver converts that toxic ammonia to a chemical called urea, which your kidneys pull out of your bloodstream to get rid of in your urine. So, as you can see, the more protein you eat, the more nitrogen your body has to clear and the more stress and strain you put on your kidneys and liver. It's like trying to dance a 2-hour routine with a sprained ankle and worn-out shoes.

This process is also dehydrating; the more water required to get rid of the nitrogen, the more minerals (like calcium) you lose. That's why high-protein diets have been linked to osteoporosis, or weakened bone—the last thing a dancer needs!

Okay, now let's tackle the protein/muscle myth. This is the one that says that if you're building up muscle, you need additional protein. I don't personally agree with this. If you're getting adequate calories to cover your energy costs, you don't need to add protein. There's also no evidence that high protein levels improve your athletic performance. Plus, the extra protein can promote dehydration, bone loss, and even add extra pounds.

So here's the three-step routine I want you to remember when it comes to protein:

Step 1: Balance your protein with other nutrients, i.e., forget about a "high-protein" diet.

Step 2: Aim for low-fat protein. This would be whole grains and beans, soy products, fish, poultry, and lean meats like pork. Personally, I stay away from red meat. I don't need the high levels of saturated fat, and it just doesn't feel good for me. And don't forget about veggies; they're protein powerhouses, too. In fact, did you know that calorie for calorie, broccoli has twice as many grams of protein as steak?

Step 3: Have a little protein with every meal and snack. Protein empties slowly from the stomach, so it keeps you feeling full longer.

Choreographer's Command #4:
Load Up on Fruits and Veggies

Quick. How many fruits or vegetables did you have yesterday (and no, French fries don't count)? That's what I thought. When it comes to fruits and vegetables, we're all—including the best dancers I know—woefully behind on what we should be getting.

You've heard about the Five-a-Day Campaign—you know, get at least five servings of fruits and vegetables a day. It sounds nearly impossible. But, as you know by now, impossible is just not in my vocabulary, whether it's pulling a complex dance step out of a singer who is sure she can't dance or getting you to eat five or more servings of fruits or vegetables a day.

Really, it's not that hard if you think about it. For instance, if you started every meal with a fruit or vegetable—a salad, a bowl of vegetable soup, a plate of sliced strawberries sprinkled with blueberries—you'd not only eat less overall, but you'd also be sneaking in that all-important fiber along with complex carbs without even trying.

Just as important, fruits and vegetables are packed with valuable micronutrients—vitamins, minerals, and plant-based chemicals called phytonutrients—that are behind the amazing ability of these foods to help prevent everything from cancer to the most common cause of blindness—macular degeneration.

If the thought of getting five servings a day (nine are better) makes you gag, however, do what I've taught you to do in Rock Your Body: break it down.

Along that route, here are the three basic steps to getting more fruits and vegetables—the rock star way.

Step 1: Start the right way. Make sure every meal—including breakfast—contains some form of fruit or vegetable. It could be a salad, a plate of fruit, or a sliced pear with a bit of cheese.

Step 2: Pump up the volume. For instance, if you're making a plate of pasta with tomato sauce (by the way, that tomato sauce counts as a veggie serving), add some grated carrots, chunked zucchini, and sliced mushrooms to that sauce. Having a spinach salad for lunch? Toss in a diced apple, a handful of raisins, and a drained can of mandarin oranges.

Step 3: Snack on them. How about dipping carrots into low-fat ranch dressing or spreading a tablespoon of peanut butter on a celery stick or an apple?

Put these three steps together and I guarantee you'll get *more* than five servings a day!

Choreographer's Command #5: Get the Right Supplements

Before we talk about vitamins and minerals, let's take a minute to talk about oxidation and antioxidants. Every time you breathe, eat, exercise, or even just move, your cells release by-products of their energy use called free radicals. I like to think of free radicals as rogue molecules. They're deformed—missing an electron—and so they bop around your body trying to steal electrons from healthy molecules, wreaking havoc in the process. Intense workouts like the Rock Your Body workout can release even more free radicals.

When other cells are damaged, your body gets a signal that it's under attack, and sends in immune system cells to repair the damage. This is good if you've cut your finger; not so good if all you did was digest a hot dog. That's because the immune response triggers inflammation. You know inflammation as the redness, swelling, and warmth you feel when a cut heals. Inside your body, however, this inflammation can cause serious damage, including heart disease and arthritis. That's why, as you'll see in this Command, getting plenty of antioxidants from food (fruits and vegetables are your best sources) *and* a good multivitamin/mineral supplement is so important. These antioxidants neutralize those rogue free radicals so they can't do any damage.

Supplement One: Multivitamin with minerals

Did you take your vitamin today? Well, what are you waiting for? I don't care how well you're eating, there's nothing wrong with a little insurance, right? Plus, as you integrate the Rock Your Body workout into your daily life, you *will* add stress to your body in the form of the additional physical activity. So the extra antioxidants in a daily vitamin can help tone down some of the negative effects from that physical stress. Hey, you're a rock star now—you've got to protect your investment, i.e., your body!

After Your "Rock Your Body" Workout . . .

I want you to slowly eat an ounce of dark—not milk—chocolate. Why? Because dark chocolate is one of the richest sources of antioxidants around—10 times more than even strawberries! This luscious, creamy, sweet source of antioxidants will help quench those damaging free radicals unleashed during your workout. Plus, it's a great motivator to get you doing the workout in the first place!

But whether it's chocolate or a piece of fruit, I do want you to have something to eat about 40 minutes after your workout to replenish your fuel supply. This is also when your body is at its peak time for absorbing the nutrients from that food. Timing your snack in this way will help reduce soreness, speed muscle repair, and replenish glucose supplies.

Also, these days even big-time doctors at places like Harvard recommend a daily multivitamin to help prevent chronic diseases, admitting that few of us get the right amount of vitamins and minerals in our diets.

That's not to say that a multivitamin or other vitamin or mineral supplements can take the place of food. "Food first," says Debra Wein, and she's absolutely right. For instance, your body might not be absorbing the full amount in the supplement, or, if you take certain supplements together—like iron and calcium—they compete for absorption in your body, so you don't get the full benefit of either.

Having said that, there are certain nutrients that women, particularly dancers and other women athletes, tend to be deficient in. One is zinc. Less than 20 percent of women get the recommended intake of zinc (8 milligrams), which is critical for building and repairing muscle tissue and producing energy. Good sources of zinc include nuts, some seafood, whole grains, fortified breakfast cereals, and dairy. Ironically, however, another nutrient found in breads, cereals, and beans called phytates can interfere with your body's absorption of zinc! So just for the insurance, make sure your multivitamin/mineral supplement contains at least 8 milligrams of this important mineral. There's no reason, however, to take a separate zinc supplement.

Another must-have is iron. Premenopausal women run a high risk of iron deficiency because of the amount of blood they lose through their periods. But as a rock star, you also lose iron through your sweat and through something called foot strike, particularly prevalent in dancers. What happens is that the constant pounding of your feet on the floor can break down red blood cells, putting you at higher risk of anemia. Debra says she sees many dancers with low iron midway through the ballet season because of this.

So choose a multivitamin with 18 milligrams of iron—no more. And ask your

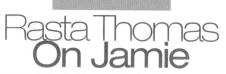

Rasta Thomas
On Jamie

Rasta is the star of the hit Twyla Tharp/Billy Joel Broadway musical *Movin' Out*.
"Jamie King is one of the most influential director/choreographers in the world. His impact on pop culture is tremendous and his dance fitness program is certain to rock your body."

doctor to test your hemoglobin levels once a year. Hemoglobin is the protein that allows your red blood vessels to carry oxygen; low levels can lead to anemia.

Other important nutrients in that multivitamin for a dancer like you include vitamin B_{12}, which tends to be low in vegetarian diets because it's found only in foods from animals (meat, eggs, and dairy). Low levels are related to muscle cramps and may also lead to high blood pressure.

Supplement Two: Calcium/magnesium supplement

I also want you to take a calcium supplement with magnesium and vitamin D to keep your bones strong. Why all three? You can't get calcium into your bones, and your bones can't use the calcium that *does* get in, without the other two. Plus, many Americans don't get enough vitamin D. The best source is 15 to 30 minutes in the sun—without sunscreen. So many people in northern climes or those who spend a lot of time indoors don't get their minimum amounts, especially in winter. Plus, it's not an easy vitamin to get from your diet (unless you're really into leafy green veggies).

Aim for a calcium supplement with about 1,500 milligrams of calcium if you haven't gone through menopause, 1,200 milligrams if you have. Make sure it contains at least 200 IU of vitamin D if you're under 50, 400 IU if you're between 51 and 70, and 600 IU if you're over 70 (hey, there is *no* age limit on rock stars!). The amount of magnesium should be at least half the amount of calcium.

Supplement Three: Fish oil

The third most important supplement is one I talked about earlier—fish oil. Unless you're eating two or three servings of fish a week, I want you to take at least 1,000 milligrams of a high-quality (i.e., all impurities taken out of it) fish oil supplement. These

Eating Like a Rock Star

If you're really into the healthy diet thing, follow a macrobiotic diet like Madonna. Basically, it's an all-organic diet high in fish, whole grains, and vegetables based on the centuries-old way the Japanese eat. And it's not surprising the Japanese have one of the lowest rates of heart disease and obesity in the world!

come in gel capsules, but if they're too big to swallow, you can get fish oil in a liquid.

The more I read about this stuff, the more I'm beginning to think it's health in a pill. Not only will it keep your heart healthier, but some studies find it can also help prevent depression, dementia, and memory loss because the fatty acids in the fish oil are so important for your brain.

And, good news for my rock stars, by reducing inflammation, fish oil can help improve and prevent chronic back pain and the other aches and pains that sometimes go along with an intense workout.

Choreographer's Command #6: Eat Less More Often

This command sounds easy to follow, but I find my dancers often have a hard time with it. Basically, I want you to get rid of that three-meals-a-day rule. Instead, I want you to plan on eating every 3 to 4 hours. Obviously, if you're eating more often, you're not going to put away the same large amounts you eat during regular meals.

Instead, I want you to consider each of these "eating times" as a mini-meal. Why? Because this way you keep your body fueled throughout the day rather than swinging back and forth between hunger and fullness.

As Debra explained it to me, it means that your body doesn't have to send out a big spike of insulin to manage the large amounts of glucose that result after large meals. Instead, your body can maintain a slow but steady supply of insulin (a hormone that helps your cells use glucose). This keeps your metabolism higher, helps build lean body tissue (aka muscle!), and can even help you lose weight, or, at the very least, keep you from gaining weight. Plus, if you're not starving, you're more likely to choose healthier meal options instead of hitting the drive-thru or reaching for that bag of cookies stashed in the cabinet.

Try eating this way for about a week and I guarantee you another benefit: a better mood and more energy. Why? Well, remember what I said about your brain needing glucose 24/7 but not being able to store it? If you maintain a steady supply of glucose, your brain stays more alert because it gets a steady supply. Otherwise it's constantly ratcheting from feast to famine. It's during those famine episodes that I've seen the sweetest dancer turn into a monster, the calmest celebrity suddenly transform into devil diva mode.

Okay, you're thinking. *I'll try it, but just how am I going to get six meals into my already hectic day?*

Planning. The key is to make at least two of those mini-meals more snacklike than meal-like, i.e., something stashed in your desk drawer, something you can carry with you when you drive the kids to soccer, something you can get into you quick when you finish a Rock Your Body workout. Which brings us to Choreographer's Command #7.

Choreographer's Command #7:
Snack Right

Snacking right means being prepared so you don't reach for a candy bar or bag of chips. It means carrying healthy snacks with you, stashing them at work, and keeping the makings for them at home. Here's a list to get you started:

For the desk drawer and pantry

- Box of whole-grain crackers
- Packages of nonperishable tuna packed in water
- 3-ounce cans of chicken
- Jar of peanut butter
- Jar of nuts
- Bag of trail mix
- Energy bars (look for ones low in fat and sugar with at least 5 grams of fiber)
- Pretzels
- Bags of baked chips
- Whole-grain bread, bagels, pitas, and tortillas
- Canned fruit (in its own juice)

For the fridge

- Cut-up fruits and vegetables. If time is an issue, buy the precut fruits and veggies available at most stores or fill a salad bar container with fruits and vegetables every few days.
- Berries (blueberries, strawberries, raspberries)
- Grapes

- Low-fat ranch dressing (for dipping aforementioned veggies)
- Hummus
- Fat-free cream cheese
- Fat-free feta cheese
- Low-fat cheese slices
- Flaxseed
- Low-fat, low-sugar yogurt (top it with a handful of flaxseeds or chopped almonds)
- Fat-free or skim cottage cheese
- Cheese sticks
- Cooked, peeled shrimp
- Turkey slices
- Precooked chicken strips
- Hard-boiled eggs
- Single-serving soups

The golden rule here is to make sure that every snack contains three things:

- A carbohydrate
- A protein
- A fruit or vegetable

Here are some easy snack combinations:

- Baby carrots dipped in hummus
- Whole-grain crackers spread thinly with peanut butter and sprinkled with raisins
- Apple slices spread with peanut butter
- Whole-wheat tortilla rolled up around 2 tablespoons of cottage cheese sprinkled with 1 ounce feta cheese. Serve with a handful of grapes.
- A pita stuffed with two precooked chicken strips, lettuce, tomato, and salsa
- Tuna spread on one slice of whole-grain bread topped with sliced cucumbers
- A hard-boiled egg and broccoli dipped in ranch dressing
- Baked corn chips with shredded low-fat cheese, melted, with salsa
- English muffin topped with cottage cheese and tomato

Break down the word *breakfast* and you get "break" and "fast." Which is literally what you're doing when you eat your toast and cereal in the morning. By the time you wake up, your body has gone between 8 and 12 hours without any food, depending on whether you're a before-bed-snack kind of person or not. Your poor body is starving. If you don't feed it soon, it's going to start literally eating itself—beginning with your rock-star muscles.

Yet about one-third of Americans skip breakfast every morning, most because they think they don't have time for it. I wonder what they'd do if they learned that consistently skipping breakfast slows their metabolisms to the point that they burn between 100 and 200 fewer calories a day; that every study on weight loss finds successful dieters always eat breakfast; and that skipping breakfast makes it more likely they'll reach for a doughnut or candy bar around 10:00 a.m., instead of one of the healthier snacks I've outlined above.

If you skip breakfast, you're also less likely to get valuable micronutrients such as folate, vitamin C, calcium, magnesium, iron, potassium, and fiber.

When I say eat breakfast, I'm not talking about two eggs over easy, country ham, buttered toast, hash browns, juice, and coffee. (Okay, the coffee can stay!)

I'm talking about things like real oatmeal sweetened with honey and sprinkled with raisins and almonds; a bowl of high-fiber, low-sugar cereal topped with sliced strawberries; a smoothie made with a banana, low-fat/low-sugar yogurt, and blueberries and sprinkled with ground flaxseeds. I'm talking about grabbing a peeled hard-boiled

The Magic of Nuts

If you've been staying away from nuts because you're worried about the calories, I've got news for you. People who snack on a handful of nuts a day—about an ounce— don't gain weight, despite the extra calories. The reason? Nuts are high in fat (but healthy fats, primarily monounsaturated), fiber, and protein—all of which are so filling you wind up eating less the rest of the day. Good options include peanuts (technically legumes, but give me a break here), walnuts, pecans, and almonds.

egg, cheese stick, and handful of grapes for the car; mixing tuna with some fat-free mayonnaise and using it to top a whole-grain English muffin.

I'm even happy to see you eat a slice of leftover pizza if it means you're eating *something*. The one thing I *don't* want to see is the sweetened-cereal-and-glass-of-orange-juice breakfast so many of us were raised on. This kind of breakfast sends a huge amount of glucose skyrocketing through your blood. But like the proverbial sprinter, that glucose will be gone within the hour, leaving you feeling more tired and hungry than before you sipped that juice and spooned in the first helping of Lucky Charms. So make sure every breakfast includes some form of protein.

I also don't like fruit juices. Even if they're unsweetened, they still pack a powerful wallop of sugar without the moderating effects of fiber. So instead of apple juice, slice up an apple. Instead of orange juice, keep a basket of clementines or navel oranges on the counter for easy peeling and eating. If you must have a glass of juice in the morning, cut it with regular or carbonated water to cut the sugar and calories in half and make sure it's calcium fortified.

Choreographer's Command #9: Drink Up!

If you can get through my Rock Your Body workout without going through at least a bottle of water, then you're not drinking enough. Come to think of it, I bet you're not drinking enough to begin with. You've undoubtedly heard the rule about eight glasses a day? Well, as a rock star, your needs are much higher. Specifically:

- Before the Rock Your Body workout, you need to prehydrate. Debra recommends 16 to 20 ounces of liquid in the 2 hours before you do the workout.
- During the workout, you need 8 ounces every 15 to 20 minutes. You can stick with water, but I really like to see my dancers with a sports drink in hand. The additional potassium, sodium, and glucose help keep your own electrolyte levels in balance and boost your energy.
- After the workout, you need to drink between 16 and 24 ounces of liquid for every pound of weight you've lost during the workout to replace fluids. Just weigh yourself before and after the workout (in dry clothing).

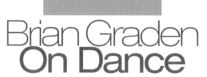

Brian Graden
On Dance

I studied music and played in bands for 10 years before joining the corporate ranks. Ultimately, I believe music is all about personal expression. The human body to me is simply one more beautiful instrument, and you can use that instrument to visually convey what you are trying to communicate. Dance allows you to say that much more. Musically, it's quite powerful.

I remember a conversation I had with a dancer, and I asked him why he chose this career. He looked at me and said, "I can't *not* dance. My body insists on dancing, my musical soul insists on moving. I don't have much of a choice." I think that if every strand of music you hear somehow inspires you to move, if it's something you just can't not do, you might as well go for it professionally as it's probably not going to go away. As for the rest of us, especially working professionals like myself, I offer this suggestion: Don't be afraid to take a page from Ellen and look silly dancing. Do it if it makes you feel good.

Brian Graden is president of Entertainment, MTV Music Group, and president of Logo Network.

If water isn't your thing (hey, some people don't like the way it "tastes"), you have other options. My favorite is iced green tea. I like to think of it as a magic elixir. Green tea is chock-full of antioxidants, which is why studies find it can help reduce the pain from inflammatory diseases like rheumatoid arthritis. It also contains huge amounts of the same heart-healthy chemical that gives red wine its magic properties: resveratrol. (You probably heard about a big study out of Harvard finding that resveratrol can also lengthen your life—even if you're overweight.) Other studies link green tea to a reduced risk of certain cancers, particularly esophageal cancer, and find it can prevent blood clots.

The one downside to green tea is that it's high in caffeine. So look for decaffeinated green tea. If you can't find it, just switch to a decaffeinated drink after 2:00 p.m., so the caffeine doesn't affect your sleep.

Most dancers I know are coffee fiends. That's fine, but if you have to say more than three words when you order your coffee from the barista, chances are you're getting a heap of extra calories with that hot drink. Forget the frappes, lattes, -chinos, etc. Stick with the real thing—a cup of coffee! Doctor it up with sugar or non-sugar sweeteners, but lighten it with fat-free milk, not cream.

As for soda, I'm going to say no. Have you ever tried to complete a jump when you've just drunk a soda? It's not pretty. Plus, there's simply nothing good about soda—at all. I mean, even coffee has been shown to reduce the risk of diabetes. But soda . . . all it's good for is leaching calcium and other minerals from your bones, contributing to ulcers, making you fat, and causing burps.

Which brings us back to water. I drink water all day long. I'm never without a water bottle, and you shouldn't be either. Beyond water bottles, here are some tips for staying hydrated:

- Fill a 1-gallon pitcher every morning for the fridge, then pour until it's gone.
- Keep half-filled bottles of water in the freezer, then top with fresh water just before you leave home to run errands.
- Drink water with all meals.
- For every alcoholic drink you down (alcohol is dehydrating), drink a full glass of water.

Choreographer's Command #10: Eat the Rock Star Way

Do you have the TV on when you're eating? Eat standing up at the sink? Eat everything on your plate? Then you've already got three strikes against you when it comes to eating the rock star way.

Now, I'm not going to hold myself up as the paragon of great dining habits. I'm on the road *100+* days a year, and I'm a terrible cook. But between my own reading and talking with Debra, I've learned a thing or two about the right way to eat so you don't inadvertently pack on the pounds. Some of them seem like common sense, others are clearly proven through research. Here are my top five:

1. **Eat the best food you can find.** That means organic fruits and vegetables, free-range chickens, antibiotic-free livestock. If you think the taste difference isn't

worth the extra price, just try a side-by-side comparison. The freshness comes through in the taste. I'm a big believer that the better something tastes, the less of it you need to eat. That's because the taste is so intense it will satisfy all your senses—including your sense of hunger—long before you can overeat.

2. **Eat slowly and with focus.** It really does take about 20 minutes for a signal of fullness to travel from your stomach to your brain. But if you eat in front of the TV, while reading, or standing over the sink, you're not paying attention to what you're eating or how you feel, just shoveling it in to clear your plate.

3. **Watch your portions.** There's no doubt that we've become a super-sizing nation. Just consider that what today passes as a "child-size" hamburger at fast food restaurants used to be a regular burger that assuaged the hunger of most adults. Today, everything is bigger, super, giant! Yet, Debra told me, studies find that we tend to eat what we're given. In other words, if you get a super large container of popcorn at the movies, you'll finish it. But if you get a small container of popcorn, you'll also eat it and feel just as satisfied. All of which just goes to disprove the statement that our eyes are bigger than our stomachs; in reality, our eyes determine the size of our stomachs.

4. **Eat at home.** The more you eat out, the more calories—and the fewer fruits and vegetables—you'll consume. That's why I order salads, eat sushi, and choose vegetable stir-fries at the Chinese food court when I'm in yet another airport. Another tip Debra recommended when eating out that I try to follow is to ask the waiter to put half your meal into a doggie bag even before it gets to your table.

5. **Go for high volume, low calories.** If you think losing weight means toddler-size portions and constant hunger, you haven't heard of "volumetrics," the nutritional finding that we're going to eat a certain volume of food regardless of the calories involved. So, for instance, if I put a small piece of steak and a few potatoes on your plate, you'll go back for seconds; but if I fill your plate with a salad, you will likely be satisfied when you finish—even though the salad might have fewer calories than the steak and fries.

How does this work in real life? Try pumping up the volume on your favorite foods. For instance, add cut-up veggies to pasta sauce to increase the volume; you'll eat less and get fewer calories. If you're eating out, order a large bowl of soup (not cream-based) as an appetizer instead of the spring rolls. Choose stew over steak, casserole over chicken breast, popcorn over potato chips. You get the picture?

Rehearsal Time

Okay, I know I've given you a lot of steps here. So let's review:

1. Choose complex carbs low on the glycemic scale and filled with fiber and whole grains.
2. Cut back on saturated fat, cut out the trans fats, and choose healthier, mono-unsaturated fats like olive oil and essential fatty acids, found in fish and flax-seed.
3. Choose lean proteins like fish, chicken, and beans, and don't overdo the protein.
4. Get at least five fruits and/or vegetables a day (nine is better).
5. Take a multivitamin/mineral supplement, a calcium/magnesium supplement with vitamin D, and a fish oil supplement (unless you're getting at least two servings of a fatty fish per week).
6. Eat more smaller meals throughout the day rather than three big ones.
7. Mix protein, carb, and fruit and/or vegetable for healthy snacks.
8. Eat breakfast every day.
9. Drink water throughout the day, including during workouts.
10. Eat the rock star way!

In the next chapter, you'll get the recipes to turn the Dancer's Diet into *your* diet.

The joy of **obstacles**—
an **opportunity** to **grow.**

Chapter 10
The Dancer's Diet Recipes

Now that you know how to eat, I've made meal planning easy on you by providing you with the 44 recipes in this chapter. They've all been chosen to support the 10 Commands of the Dancer's Diet, and all are designed to improve your health, stamina, and (if you need it) weight if you incorporate them into an overall healthy diet.

You don't have to stick to these recipes as you transform your nutritional habits to the 10 Commands, but I recommend you choose at least one recipe a day to try. I guarantee it will help you reach your dietary goals.

Snacks and Smoothies
Veggie Pizza 225 Calories

Prep time: 10 minutes; Cook time: 3 minutes

1 English muffin, split

¼ cup (60 ml) tomato sauce

¼ cup (4 tablespoons) chopped mushrooms

2 tablespoons chopped green bell pepper

2 tablespoons chopped onion

2 tablespoons shredded reduced-fat mozzarella cheese

Preheat the oven or toaster oven to 350°F (180°C).

Toast the muffin halves. Evenly divide the sauce, mushrooms, pepper, onion, and cheese between the muffin halves.

Bake for 3 minutes, or until the cheese is melted.

Makes 1 serving

PER SERVING: 225 calories, 10 g protein, 41 g carbohydrates, 3 g fat, 6 mg cholesterol, 717 mg sodium, 4 g fiber

Cottage Cheese Dill Dip 20 Calories

Prep time: 5 minutes

1 cup (230 g) fat-free cottage cheese

¼ teaspoon onion powder

½ teaspoon garlic salt

1 teaspoon chopped fresh dillweed, or ½ teaspoon dried dillweed

In a food processor, combine the cottage cheese, onion powder, garlic salt, and dillweed. Pulse until smooth, about 30 seconds.

Serve as dip for raw vegetables or fat-free tortilla chips.

Makes 8 servings, 2 tablespoons each (1 cup)

PER SERVING: 20 calories, 3 g protein, 2 g carbohydrates, 0 g fat, 1 mg cholesterol, 170 mg sodium, 0 g fiber

Apple-Cinnamon Yogurt 229 Calories

Prep time: 5 minutes

1 small apple, cored and chopped

2 tablespoons chopped walnuts

1 teaspoon honey (optional)

⅛ teaspoon ground cinnamon

½ cup (115 g) fat-free plain yogurt

Place the apple and walnuts in a microwaveable bowl. Top with the honey, if using, and cinnamon. Microwave on high power for 1 minute, or until warmed. Top with the yogurt.

Makes 1 serving

PER SERVING: 229 calories, 7 g protein, 34 g carbohydrates, 10 g fat, 5 mg cholesterol, 70 mg sodium, 6 g fiber

Strawberry-Banana Popsicles 45 Calories

Prep time: 5 minutes; Freeze time: 3 hours

1 cup (240 ml) water
1 cup (240 ml) fat-free milk
15 strawberries, sliced
2 ripe bananas, sliced
1 tablespoon honey

In a blender, combine the ingredients. Blend for about 3 minutes, or until smooth. Pour the mixture into a popsicle mold, and freeze for at least 3 hours.

Makes 10 popsicles

PER SERVING: 45 calories, 1 g protein, 11 g carbohydrates, 0 g fat, .5 mg cholesterol, 11 mg sodium, 2 g fiber

Fruity Health Smoothie 330 Calories

Prep time: 7 minutes

1 bag (16 ounces) (450 g) frozen peach slices
1 can (16 ounces) (450 g) mandarin oranges, drained
1 can (16 ounces) (450 g) apricots, drained
¼ cup (4 tablespoons) oat bran
Pinch of nutmeg
1 cup (240 ml) light coconut milk

In a blender, combine the peaches, oranges, apricots, oat bran, and nutmeg. Blend until smooth. Add the coconut milk and blend until combined. Serve over ice.

Makes 4 servings

PER SERVING: 330 calories, 5 g protein, 56 g carbohydrates, 13 g fat, 0 mg cholesterol, 17 mg sodium, 9 g fiber

Mango Freeze 122 Calories

Prep time: 5 minutes

½ cup (120 ml) vanilla soy milk

¼ cup (60 ml) cold water

1 cup (150 g) frozen mango

½ banana

½ cup (75 g) fresh or frozen blueberries

In a blender, combine the soy milk, water, mango, banana, and blueberries. Blend for 1 minute, then stir. Repeat once or twice, depending on the density of the frozen mango.

Makes 2 servings

PER SERVING: 122 calories, 3 g protein, 28 g carbohydrates, 2 g fat, 0 mg cholesterol, 11 mg sodium, 4 g fiber

Tea Frosty 92 Calories

Prep time: 5 minutes

3 or 4 ice cubes

1 cup (240 ml) brewed black or green tea

1 cup (150 g)low-fat vanilla ice cream or ice milk

In a blender, combine the ice cubes, tea, and ice cream or ice milk. Blend until smooth.

Makes 2 servings

PER SERVING: 92 calories, 3 g protein, 15 g carbohydrates, 3 g fat, 9 mg cholesterol, 56 mg sodium, 0 g fiber

Kitchen Tip
You can add a little Splenda to this recipe if it's not sweet enough for you.

Black Bean Salsa 17 Calories

Prep time: 12 minutes; Stand time: 30 minutes

1 can (14½ ounces) (400 g) black beans, drained
3 medium tomatoes, diced
2 tablespoons frozen orange juice concentrate
½ cup (15 g) chopped cilantro
Salt

In a medium bowl, mix the beans, tomatoes, orange juice concentrate, and cilantro. Add salt to taste. Let the mixture stand for 30 minutes to allow the flavors to combine.

Makes 28 servings (3½ cups)

PER SERVING: 17 calories, 1 g protein, 3 g carbohydrates, 0 g fat, 0 mg cholesterol, 40 mg sodium, 1 g fiber

Pineapple Salsa 16 Calories

Prep time: 5 minutes; Stand time: 30 minutes

1 jalapeño chile pepper, chopped (wear plastic gloves when handling)
1 cup (180 g) chopped pineapple
2 tablespoons chopped fresh cilantro
1 red onion, chopped
Juice of 1 lime

In a small bowl, combine the jalapeño, pineapple, cilantro, and onion, then add the lime juice. Let stand for 30 minutes to allow the flavors to blend.

Makes 8 servings

PER SERVING: 16 calories, 0 g protein, 4 g carbohydrates, 0 g fat, 0 mg cholesterol, 1 mg sodium, 1 g fiber

Breakfast
Spinach Omelets 249 Calories

Prep time: 5 minutes; Cook time: 7 minutes

4 large eggs

4 egg whites

1 tablespoon 1 percent milk

1 teaspoon trans-free margarine or butter

1½ cups (45 g) loosely packed baby spinach

¼ cup (about 1 ounce) (about 30 g) shredded part-skim mozzarella or reduced-fat Cheddar cheese

Salt

Ground black pepper

In a medium bowl, beat the whole eggs, egg whites, and milk. In a large skillet over medium heat, melt the margarine or butter. Add the beaten egg mixture and cook until it begins to set. Sprinkle the spinach and cheese on top, cook for 1 to 2 minutes longer, then gently fold into an omelet. Cook until the spinach appears wilted and the eggs are completely set. Season with salt and pepper to taste and serve immediately.

Makes 2 servings

PER SERVING: 249 calories, 23 g protein, 4 g carbohydrates, 15 g fat, 438 mg cholesterol, 368 mg sodium, 1 g fiber

Kitchen Tip
To prevent your omelet from getting tough and chewy, bring the eggs to room temperature before adding them to the pan. Cold eggs take longer to cook through.
Also, make sure the pan is well-heated before adding the eggs.

Southwestern Frittata 81 Calories

Prep time: 10 minutes; Cook time: 20 minutes

1 tablespoon olive oil

1 green bell pepper, diced

1 sweet onion, diced

4 Roma tomatoes, diced

4 eggs, lightly beaten

Salt

Ground black pepper

Preheat the oven to 350°F (180°C).

In a medium oven-safe, nonstick skillet, heat the oil over medium heat. Add the bell pepper and onion, and cook for 5 minutes, or until the onion is translucent. Add the tomatoes and eggs. Stir constantly until the eggs are distributed all over the bottom of the pan. Cook for 1 to 2 minutes, or until the eggs begin to set. Season with salt and black pepper to taste.

Bake in the oven for 10 minutes, or until the eggs are cooked and the mixture has puffed slightly. Let the frittata cool slightly and cut it into wedges for serving.

Makes 4 servings

PER SERVING: 81 calories, 5 g protein, 8 g carbohydrates, 4 g fat, 0 mg cholesterol, 60 mg sodium, 2 g fiber

Scrambled Egg Wrap 274 Calories

Prep time: 5 minutes; Cook time: 5 minutes

2 eggs, lightly beaten

2 tablespoons herb cream cheese spread

1 whole wheat flour tortilla

2 tablespoons low-fat grated Cheddar cheese

½ tablespoon chopped fresh basil

½ tablespoon chopped fresh chives

1 tablespoon salsa

Preheat the oven to warm. Coat a small skillet with cooking spray. Add the eggs to the skillet and cook for 2 minutes, stirring constantly. Spread the cheese spread on the wrap, then add the eggs, cheese, basil, chives, and salsa. Roll up the wrap, folding in the sides, and heat it in the oven for 3 minutes, or until warmed through.

Makes 1 serving

PER SERVING: 274 calories, 20 g protein, 22 g carbohydrates, 14 g fat, 436 mg cholesterol, 504 mg sodium, 2 g fiber

Baked Apple Oatmeal 298 Calories

Prep time: 5 minutes; Cook time: 15–20 minutes

1 medium cooking apple, cored and chopped

½ cup (30 g) old-fashioned rolled oats

2 tablespoons raisins

½ teaspoon cinnamon

Pinch of salt

1 cup (240 ml) water

Preheat the oven to 350°F (180°C).

In a small baking dish, combine the apple, oats, raisins, cinnamon, salt, and water and stir well.

Bake, uncovered, stirring once or twice, for 15 to 20 minutes, or until the mixture becomes thick and the apple pieces are fork-tender.

Makes 1 serving

PER SERVING: 298 calories, 7 g protein, 66 g carbohydrates, 3 g fat, 0 mg cholesterol, 4 mg sodium, 11 g fiber

Hearty Waffles 370 Calories

Prep time: 15 minutes; Chill time: 30 minutes; Cook time: 10 minutes

½ cup (30 g) quick-cooking oatmeal

¼ cup (4 tablespoons) oat bran

2 tablespoons whole wheat flour

2 tablespoons unbleached or all-purpose flour

1½ tablespoons packed brown sugar

1 tablespoon ground cinnamon

½ teaspoon ground nutmeg

1¼ cups (300 ml) fat-free milk

1 tablespoon canola oil

2 tablespoons lite blueberry or maple syrup

½ cup (75 g) blueberries

In a large bowl, combine the oatmeal, oat bran, whole wheat flour, all-purpose flour, brown sugar, cinnamon, and nutmeg. Add the milk and oil and stir to combine. Refrigerate for 30 minutes, or until the batter is thickened.

Preheat a waffle iron according to the manufacturer's directions. Pour the batter onto the waffle iron (amount will vary according to manufacturer) and cook for 5 minutes, or until golden brown. Serve topped with the syrup and blueberries.

Makes 2 waffles

PER WAFFLE: 370 calories, 13 g protein, 64 g carbohydrates, 10 g fat, 5 mg cholesterol, 290 mg sodium, 8 g fiber

Oatmeal and Wheat Maple Muffins 94 Calories

Prep time: 18 minutes; Cook time: 20 minutes

1 cup (125 g) all-purpose flour

¾ cup (90 g) whole wheat flour

¾ cup (45 g) rolled oats

2 teaspoons baking powder

2 teaspoons ground cinnamon

1 teaspoon ground nutmeg

½ teaspoon baking soda

½ teaspoon salt

½ teaspoon cloves

1 cup (240 g) unsweetened applesauce

1 cup (230 g) fat-free plain yogurt

½ cup (120 ml) maple syrup

½ cup (110 g) packed dark brown sugar

¼ cup (60 g) reduced-fat sour cream

1 egg or ¼ cup (60 ml) egg substitute

2 teaspoons vanilla extract

Preheat the oven to 375°F (190°C). Coat two 12-cup muffin pans with cooking spray.

In a large bowl, combine the flours, oats, baking powder, cinnamon, nutmeg, baking soda, salt, and cloves.

In a medium bowl, combine the applesauce, yogurt, syrup, sugar, sour cream, egg or egg substitute, and vanilla extract. Add to the flour mixture and stir just until blended. Evenly divide the batter among the prepared muffin cups.

Bake for 20 minutes, or until a wooden pick inserted in the center of a muffin comes out clean. Cool on a rack.

Makes 24 muffins

PER MUFFIN: 94 calories, 2 g protein, 20 g carbohydrates, 1 g fat, 10 mg cholesterol, 128 mg sodium, 1 g fiber

High-Fiber Raisin Bran Muffins 122 Calories

Prep time: 15 minutes; Bake time: 30–35 minutes; Cool time: 10 minutes

1 cup (125 g) whole wheat pastry flour

¼ cup (30 g) unbleached or all-purpose flour

2 teaspoons baking soda

¼ teaspoon salt

½ cup (125 g) applesauce

1 teaspoon vanilla extract

1 egg + 1 egg white

1 apple, chopped

⅓ cup (20 g) quick-cooking oats

1 teaspoon cinnamon

⅓ cup (75 g) brown sugar

1 cup (240 ml) skim milk

2 cups (100 g) raisin bran cereal

Preheat the oven to 350°F (180°C). Line a 12-cup muffin pan with paper muffin cups.

In a large mixing bowl, combine the flours, baking soda, and salt. Add the applesauce, vanilla, egg and egg white, apple, oats, cinnamon, and brown sugar. Stir well. In a small bowl, mix together the milk and cereal and let stand for a few minutes. Add the cereal and milk mixture to the apple mixture and stir until just blended. Spoon the mixture into each muffin cup, filling each cup about three-quarters full.

Bake for 30 to 35 minutes, or until a wooden pick inserted in the center of a muffin comes out clean. Cool on a rack for 10 minutes before serving.

Makes 12 muffins

PER MUFFIN: 122 calories, 4 g protein, 26 g carbohydrates, 1 g fat, 18 mg cholesterol, 221 mg sodium, 3 g fiber

Lunch
Thai Squash Soup 92 Calories

Prep time: 10 minutes; Cook time: 20 minutes

5 or 6 shallots, unpeeled

1 can (13½ ounces) (400 ml) light coconut milk

2 cups (480 ml) reduced-sodium chicken broth

1½ pounds (680 g) butternut squash, peeled and cut into ½" cubes

½ cup (20 g) packed fresh cilantro plus 1 tablespoon chopped, for garnish

½ teaspoon salt

2 tablespoons fish sauce

¼ cup (4 tablespoons) minced scallions, green parts only

Ground black pepper

Preheat the broiler. Spray a sheet of heavy foil with cooking spray and place the shallots on top. When the broiler is ready, broil the shallots, turning occasionally, for about 5 to 7 minutes, or until softened and blackened. Remove from the broiler, let cool, then peel and halve them lengthwise.

In a large pot over medium-high heat, combine the shallots, coconut milk, broth, squash, and ½ cup of cilantro. Cook just until the mixture begins to boil. Reduce the heat, add the salt, and simmer for about 10 minutes, or until the squash is tender. Stir in the fish sauce and cook for 2 to 3 minutes longer.

Garnish each serving with a sprinkling of the minced scallion greens and the chopped cilantro and season with pepper to taste.

Makes 6 (1-cup) servings

PER SERVING: 92 calories, 4 g protein, 20 g carbohydrates, 1 g fat, 1 mg cholesterol, 728 mg sodium, 2 g fiber

Long-Grain Rice and Lentil Soup 130 Calories

Prep time: 15 minutes; Cook time: 45 minutes

5 cans (14½ ounces each) (400 ml each) reduced-sodium chicken broth

1½ cups (300 g) lentils, rinsed and drained

1 cup (180 g) long-grain brown rice

2 cans (14½ ounces each) (400 g each) diced tomatoes

3 carrots, chopped

1 small onion, chopped

1 rib celery, chopped

3 cloves garlic, minced

1 teaspoon dried basil

1 teaspoon dried oregano

1 teaspoon dried thyme

1 bay leaf

2 tablespoons cider vinegar

½ cup (30 g) finely chopped fresh parsley

Ground black pepper

In a large pot over medium-high heat, combine the broth, lentils, rice, tomatoes (with juice), carrots, onion, celery, garlic, basil, oregano, thyme, and bay leaf. Bring to a boil, then reduce the heat to low. Simmer, covered, for 45 minutes, stirring occasionally. Remove from the heat and add the vinegar, parsley, and pepper to taste. Remove and discard the bay leaf, adjust the seasonings, and serve.

Makes 16 (1-cup) servings

PER SERVING: 130 calories, 7 g protein, 24 g carbohydrates, 1 g fat, 1 mg cholesterol, 34 mg sodium, 7 g fiber

Hearty Veggie Stew 330 Calories

Prep time: 15 minutes; Cook time: 1 hour, 10 minutes

3 tablespoons olive oil

1 medium yellow or white onion, coarsely chopped

½ teaspoon salt

2 cloves garlic, minced

6 russet potatoes, quartered

1 pound (450 g) carrots, cleaned and cut into thirds

1 can (14½ ounces) (400 ml) low-sodium vegetable broth

½ cup (120 ml) ketchup

1 package (10 ounces) (300 g) frozen green beans, thawed

1 package (10 ounces) (300 g) frozen green peas, thawed

1 cup (145 g) dried, sliced shiitake mushrooms

2 tablespoons Worcestershire sauce

1 tablespoon dried oregano

½ teaspoon ground black pepper

½ teaspoon red-pepper flakes

Warm the oil in a large pot over medium heat. When hot, add the onion and salt and cook for 5 minutes, or until soft. Add the garlic and cook for 2 minutes longer, until lightly browned. Add the potatoes, carrots, broth, and ketchup and cook, uncovered and stirring occasionally, just until boiling. Reduce the heat to low and add the green beans, peas, mushrooms, and Worcestershire sauce. Stir in the oregano, black pepper, and red-pepper flakes and simmer, uncovered, for 30 minutes, or until the potatoes and carrots are tender.

Makes 6 (1-cup) servings

PER SERVING: 330 calories, 9 g protein, 62 g carbohydrates, 8 g fat, 0 mg cholesterol, 720 mg sodium, 10 g fiber

Turkey Chili · 220 Calories

Prep time: 10 minutes; Cook time: 40 minutes

2 tablespoons vegetable oil

1 large onion, chopped

1 green bell pepper, chopped

1 red bell pepper, chopped

3 cloves garlic, minced

1 teaspoon to 1 tablespoon chili powder

1 tablespoon ground cumin

1 pound (450 g) lean ground turkey breast

2 cans (14½ ounces each) (400 g each) pinto beans, rinsed and drained

2 cans (14½ ounces each) (400 g each) diced tomatoes

1 small bunch cilantro, stemmed and chopped

Juice of ½ lime

Salt

Ground black pepper

Warm the oil in a large pot over medium heat. When hot, add the onion and bell peppers and cook for 5 to 10 minutes, or until soft. Add the garlic, chili powder, and cumin and cook, stirring, for 2 to 3 minutes. Add the turkey and cook, stirring, until no longer pink. Add the beans and tomatoes (with juice) and bring to a boil. Reduce the heat and simmer, uncovered, for about 20 minutes. Stir in the cilantro and lime juice and season with salt and black pepper to taste.

Makes 6 (1½-cup) servings

PER SERVING: 220 calories, 5 g protein, 82 g carbohydrates, 7 g fat, 2 mg cholesterol, 60 mg sodium, 21 g fiber

Steak Salad 303 Calories

Prep time: 10 minutes; Marinate time: 30 minutes; Cook time: 10 minutes

2 tablespoons light soy sauce

1 clove garlic, minced

6 ounces (170 g) beef tenderloin, thinly sliced

2 teaspoons toasted sesame oil

¼ cup (60 ml) reduced-fat beef broth

1 medium red bell pepper, sliced

½ onion, sliced into rings

½ pound (230 g) mushrooms of your choice, sliced

½ head leaf lettuce, washed and torn into bite-size pieces

In a shallow glass dish, mix the soy sauce and garlic. Lay the beef slices in the sauce and turn several times to coat. Cover and refrigerate for at least 30 minutes, or overnight.

Warm the oil in a large skillet or wok over medium-high heat. When hot, add the beef and its marinade and cook, stirring constantly, for 5 minutes, or until no longer pink. Transfer the beef to a large bowl and set aside. Add the broth to the skillet and cook with the pepper, onion, and mushrooms for about 1 minute, or until the vegetables are bright and crisp-tender.

In a large bowl, toss the vegetables and beef with the lettuce and serve.

Makes 2 servings

PER SERVING: 303 calories, 31 g protein, 17 g carbohydrates, 13 g fat, 71 mg cholesterol, 687 mg sodium, 4 g fiber

Spinach and Chickpea Salad 370 Calories

Prep time: 5 minutes

1 bag (6 ounces) (170 g) fresh baby spinach

1 can (14½ ounces) (400 g) chickpeas, drained and rinsed

¼ cup (1 ounce) (30 g) grated fat-free Parmesan cheese

½ cup (8 tablespoons) alfalfa sprouts

2 tablespoons olive oil

¼ cup (60 ml) Champagne vinegar

In a large bowl, toss together the spinach and chickpeas. Top with the cheese and sprouts. In a small bowl, whisk together the oil and vinegar and pour over the salad just before serving.

Makes 2 servings

PER SERVING: 370 calories, 14 g protein, 45 g carbohydrates, 15 g fat, 10 mg cholesterol, 620 mg sodium, 9 g fiber

Easy Pita Pockets 210 Calories

Prep time: 10 minutes

2 whole wheat pitas, halved

½ pound (230 g) cooked turkey breast, thinly sliced

1 green bell pepper, sliced

1 tomato, thinly sliced

¼ cup (1 ounce) (30 g) shredded reduced-fat Cheddar or Monterey Jack cheese

¼ cup (60 ml) light ranch salad dressing

In each pita half, place one-quarter of the turkey, a few slices of pepper and tomato, and 1 tablespoon of cheese. Top with 1 tablespoon of dressing.

Makes 4 servings

PER SERVING: 210 calories, 15 g protein, 25 g carbohydrates, 6 g fat, 25 mg cholesterol, 860 mg sodium, 3 g fiber

Turkey-Spinach Medley on Pitas 388 Calories

Prep time: 10 minutes; Cook time: 25 minutes

1–2 teaspoons olive oil

1–2 cloves garlic, minced

½ medium onion, chopped

1 pound (450 g) lean ground turkey breast

1 package (10 ounces) (300 g) frozen chopped spinach, thawed and squeezed dry

Ground black pepper

4 whole wheat pitas, halved

1 medium tomato, chopped

Warm the oil in a large skillet over medium-high heat. When hot, add the garlic and onion and cook for about 5 minutes, or until tender. Add the turkey and cook, breaking up the turkey with the back of a spoon as you stir, for 15 minutes, or until no longer pink. Add the spinach and cook for 5 to 7 minutes longer.

Season with pepper to taste and spoon equal portions into the pitas. Top with tomatoes and serve.

Makes 4 servings

PER SERVING: 388 calories, 29 g protein, 41 g carbohydrates, 13 g fat, 90 mg cholesterol, 509 mg sodium, 7 g fiber

Sweet and Spicy Warm Chicken Salad

170 Calories

Prep time: 10 minutes; Cook time: 6 minutes

2 chicken breast halves (230 g), sliced

1 small onion, diced

1 jalapeño chile pepper, sliced (wear plastic gloves when handling)

1 can (6½ ounces) (180 g) sliced mushrooms, drained

1 bag (1 pound) (450 g) baby spinach

1 cucumber, sliced

½ cup (60 g) dried orange-flavored cranberries

½ cup (15 g) fat-free croutons

Salt

Ground black pepper

½ cup (120 ml) fat-free raspberry pecan salad dressing

Coat a large nonstick saucepan with cooking spray. Add the chicken and cook on medium-high heat for 3 minutes or until the juices run clear. Remove and keep warm. Add the onion, jalapeño, and mushrooms. Cook for 3 minutes, or until brown. Mix with the chicken.

In a large bowl, combine the chicken mixture with the spinach, cucumber, cranberries, croutons, and salt and black pepper to taste. Add the dressing and toss gently to combine. Serve immediately.

Makes 6 servings

PER SERVING: 170 calories, 13 g protein, 29 g carbohydrates, 2 g fat, 23 mg cholesterol, 328 mg sodium, 6 g fiber

Wild Rice Salad 222 Calories

Prep time: 20 minutes; Cook time: 45 minutes; Chill time: 2 hours

¼ cup (30 g) almonds, pecans, walnuts, and/or cashews

1 box (4 ounces) (120 g) wild rice

3 ribs celery, chopped

1 red bell pepper, finely chopped

1 yellow bell pepper, finely chopped

1 bunch scallions, chopped

1 small red onion, chopped

¼ cup (60 ml) balsamic vinegar

2 tablespoons finely chopped fresh basil

2 tablespoons finely chopped parsley

1 tablespoon Dijon mustard

1 clove garlic, minced

½ teaspoon kosher salt

⅛ teaspoon freshly ground black pepper

⅛ teaspoon dried oregano

1 teaspoon sugar

¼ cup (60 ml) extra virgin olive oil

3 cups (100 g) assorted salad greens

Preheat the oven to 425°F (200°C).

Spread the nuts in a single layer on a baking sheet. Bake for 3 minutes, or until they begin to brown. Remove and set aside.

Prepare the wild rice according to package directions. In a large serving bowl, combine the rice, celery, bell peppers, scallions, onion, and nuts. In a measuring cup, combine the vinegar, basil, parsley, mustard, garlic, salt, black pepper, oregano, and sugar. Gradually add the oil. Stir to combine. Pour all but 2 tablespoons of the dressing over the rice mixture. Cover and refrigerate for at least 2 hours or overnight.

Serve the rice salad over the greens. Drizzle with the reserved dressing.

Makes 6 servings

PER SERVING: 222 calories, 5 g protein, 25 g carbohydrates, 12 g fat, 0 mg cholesterol, 264 mg sodium, 4 g fiber

Black Bean Quesadillas 450 Calories

Prep time: 10 minutes; Cook time: 20 minutes

1 can (14–19 ounces) (450 g) no-salt black beans, rinsed and drained

1 teaspoon dried onion flakes

8 flour or whole wheat tortillas (8" in diameter)

2 cups (8 ounces) (230 g) shredded low-fat Colby or Monterey Jack cheese

1 cup (240 ml) salsa (optional)

½ cup (115 g) fat-free sour cream (optional)

Place the beans and onion flakes in a small saucepan over low heat and cook for 5 minutes, or until warm. Mash the beans with a spoon. Keep warm.

Meanwhile, heat a large nonstick skillet coated with cooking spray over medium heat. Place 1 tortilla in the pan and sprinkle with ¼ cup of the cheese. Cook for 2 minutes, or until the cheese melts. Spoon one-quarter of the bean mixture on top and sprinkle with ¼ cup cheese. Top with another tortilla. Carefully turn the quesadilla and cook for 2 minutes, or until browned. Repeat to make a total of 4 quesadillas. Serve with the salsa and sour cream, if using.

Makes 4 quesadillas

PER QUESADILLA: 450 calories, 26 g protein, 57 g carbohydrates, 11 g fat, 10 mg cholesterol, 840 mg sodium, 3 g fiber

Portobello Burgers with Shoestring Fries 418 Calories

Fries
Prep time: 10 minutes; Cook time: 27 minutes

2 egg whites

½ teaspoon paprika

¼ teaspoon garlic powder

2 pounds (1 kg) baking potatoes, cut lengthwise into thin strips

Burgers
Prep time: 5 minutes; Cook time: 10 minutes

1 hard-cooked egg white, finely chopped

2 tablespoons fat-free mayonnaise

1 tablespoon minced shallots

1 tablespoon chili sauce

1 teaspoon sweet pickle relish

8 medium portobello mushroom caps

Salt and ground black pepper

4 whole-grain hamburger buns

4 leaves lettuce

8 tomato slices

To make the fries:

Preheat the oven to 425°F (200°C). Coat 2 baking sheets with cooking spray.

In a large bowl, combine the egg whites, paprika, and garlic powder. Add the potatoes and toss to coat. Place on the prepared baking sheets, allowing the excess egg whites to drain off. Bake for 15 minutes. Switch the position of the baking sheets and bake for 12 minutes longer, or until golden brown and crispy.

To make the burgers:

Coat a grill rack or broiler-pan rack with cooking spray. Preheat the grill or broiler.

In a small bowl, combine the egg white, mayonnaise, shallots, chili sauce, and relish. Set aside. Coat the mushroom caps with cooking spray and season with salt and pepper. Cook 4" from the heat for 4 minutes per side, or until soft and tender. If desired, lightly toast the buns on the grill or under the broiler.

Place the lettuce leaves on the bottom halves of the buns. Top each with a mushroom cap. Place 2 tomato slices on each burger, then top with a second mushroom cap. Spread the seasoned mayonnaise on the bun tops and place on the burgers. Serve with the fries.

Makes 4 servings

PER SERVING: 418 calories, 17 g protein, 80 g carbohydrates, 2 g fat, 0 mg cholesterol, 450 mg sodium, 12 g fiber

Chicken Tacos with Salsa 239 Calories

Prep time: 15 minutes; Marinate time: 1–4 hours; Cook time: 10 minutes

3 limes

¼ cup (60 ml) orange juice

¼ cup (10 g) chopped fresh cilantro

3 cloves garlic, minced

½ teaspoon ground cumin

4 boneless, skinless chicken breast halves (450 g), pounded to ½" thickness

1 large red onion, thinly sliced

6 whole wheat flour tortillas (8" diameter)

2 cups (480 ml) prepared salsa

¾ cup (180 g) fat-free sour cream

2 cups (75 g) finely shredded leaf lettuce

Grate the rind from the limes into a large bowl. Cut the limes in half and squeeze the juice into the bowl; discard the limes. Stir in the orange juice, cilantro, garlic, and cumin. Add the chicken and turn to coat. Cover and refrigerate for at least 1 hour or up to 4 hours; turn at least once while marinating.

Heat a large skillet coated with cooking spray over medium heat. Remove the chicken from the marinade; discard the marinade. Add the chicken and onion to the skillet and cook for 3 minutes per side, or until a thermometer inserted in the thickest portion registers 160°F and the juices run clear and the onions are softened. Cut the chicken into 1" slices.

Wrap the tortillas in a paper towel and microwave on high power for 1 minute. Divide the chicken mixture among the tortillas. Top with the salsa, sour cream, and lettuce. Roll to enclose the filling. Slice each taco in half.

Makes 6 tacos

PER TACO: 239 calories, 25 g protein, 37 g carbohydrates, 2 g fat, 45 mg cholesterol, 630 mg sodium, 5 g fiber

Dinner
Turkey-Mushroom Burgers 300 Calories

Prep time: 5 minutes; Cook time: 16 minutes

1 pound (450 g) lean ground turkey breast

2 cups (140 g) sliced mushrooms, divided

¼ cup (4 tablespoons) chopped fresh parsley

1½ tablespoons Worcestershire sauce

½ teaspoon onion salt

1 tablespoon vegetable oil

4 hamburger buns, split

In a large bowl, combine the turkey, 1 cup (70 g) of the mushrooms, the parsley, Worcestershire sauce, and onion salt. With clean hands, mix the ingredients until thoroughly combined and shape into 4 equal-size patties. Set aside.

Warm the oil in a large skillet over medium heat. When hot, add the remaining 1 cup (70 g) of mushrooms and cook, stirring, for 2 minutes, or until brown. Transfer the mushrooms to a plate and cover to keep warm. Place the patties in the skillet over medium heat and cook, turning occasionally, for 12 to 14 minutes, or until a thermometer inserted in the center registers 165°F and the meat is no longer pink.

Set the patties on the buns, top with the sautéed mushrooms, and serve.

Makes 4 servings

PER SERVING: 300 calories, 31 g protein, 24 g carbohydrates, 9 g fat, 80 mg cholesterol, 550 mg sodium, 4 g fiber

Kitchen Tip
Wet your hands with cold water to keep meat from sticking to them.

Mango Salsa Grouper 286 Calories

Prep time: 15 minutes; Chill time: 2 hours; Cook time: 8–10 minutes

1 mango, finely chopped

½ cup (15 g) chopped fresh cilantro

½ cup (75 g) chopped red bell pepper

½ cup (75 g) chopped poblano or green bell pepper

½ cup (75 g) chopped red onion

¼ cup (60 ml) rice wine vinegar

Salt

Ground black pepper

1–2 teaspoons olive oil

4 grouper fillets (5–6 ounces/140–170 g each)

In a medium bowl, combine the mango, cilantro, red bell pepper, poblano or green bell pepper, onion, and vinegar. Toss well and season with salt and black pepper to taste. Cover and refrigerate the mango salsa for at least 2 hours.

Preheat the grill to medium-high. Coat a piece of foil with cooking spray and lay it on a grill rack.

Rub the oil on the fish and place on the foil over the coolest part of the grill. Grill for 8 to 10 minutes, or until the fish flakes easily. Serve with the mango salsa.

Makes 4 servings

PER SERVING: 286 calories, 51 g protein, 12 g carbohydrates, 3 g fat, 0 mg cholesterol, 140 mg sodium, 2 g fiber

Tofu-Walnut Patties 170 Calories

Prep time: 25 minutes; Cook time: 10 minutes

½ pound (230 g) firm tofu

¾ cup (45 g) rolled oats

1 cup fresh whole wheat bread crumbs (from about 2 slices)

¼ cup (30 g) whole wheat flour

1 onion, chopped

½ cup (50 g) walnuts, finely chopped

1½ teaspoons beef bouillon powder

¼–½ teaspoon garlic powder

¼ teaspoon salt

2 teaspoons dried savory or 1 teaspoon dried sage

½–1 cup (120–240 ml) water

With the back of a fork, finely crumble the tofu into a large bowl. Add the oats, bread crumbs, and flour and mix gently, then add the onion, walnuts, bouillon powder, garlic powder, salt, and savory or sage and mix again. Slowly add enough water so that you can shape the tofu mixture into 6 patties.

Coat a large skillet with cooking spray and cook the patties over medium-high heat for 3 to 5 minutes, or until golden. Flip the patties and continue cooking until browned on the other side.

Makes 6 servings

PER SERVING: 170 calories, 7 g protein, 19 g carbohydrates, 8 g fat, 0 mg cholesterol, 350 mg sodium, 3 g fiber

Kitchen Tip

This recipe is also great baked! Place the patties on a baking sheet lightly coated with cooking spray and bake in a 350°F (180°C) oven for 20 minutes, turning after 10 minutes. You can also use this mixture to make meatballs.

Incredible Meat Loaf 285 Calories

Prep time: 5 minutes; Bake time: 55–65 minutes; Stand time: 10 minutes

1½ pounds (680 g) 85 percent lean ground beef

1 cup (200 g) cooked rice

2 tablespoons fat-free yogurt

1 rib celery, diced

½ medium onion, grated or diced

Salt

Ground black pepper

Preheat the oven to 350°F (180°C). Coat a baking sheet with cooking spray.

In a large mixing bowl, mix together the beef, rice, yogurt, celery, onion, and salt and pepper to taste. Form into a loaf on the prepared baking sheet.

Bake for 55 to 65 minutes, or until a thermometer inserted in the center registers 160°F and the meat is no longer pink. Let stand for 10 minutes before slicing.

Makes 6 servings

PER SERVING: 285 calories, 22 g protein, 9 g carbohydrates, 17 g fat, 78 mg cholesterol, 88 mg sodium, 1 g fiber

Salsa Chicken Stir-Fry 167 Calories

Prep time: 10 minutes; Cook time: 12 minutes

1 pound (450 g) boneless, skinless chicken breasts, cut into thin strips

½ onion, thinly sliced

1 clove garlic, minced

½ red bell pepper, thinly sliced

1 cup (70 g) broccoli florets

1 cup (240 ml) salsa

Salt

Ground black pepper

¼ teaspoon ground red pepper (optional)

In a large nonstick skillet over medium heat, cook the chicken, stirring frequently, until it is no longer pink and the juices run clear. Remove the chicken from the pan. In the same pan, cook the onion, garlic, bell pepper, and broccoli until crisp-tender. Return the chicken to the pan. Add the salsa and stir to coat. Cook for 1 to 2 minutes. Season to taste with salt, black pepper, and red pepper, if using. Serve immediately.

Makes 4 servings

PER SERVING: 167 calories, 28 g protein, 8 g carbohydrates, 2 g fat, 66 mg cholesterol, 326 mg sodium, 2 g fiber

Chunky Chicken Stew 260 Calories

Prep time: 15 minutes; Cook time: 1 hour, 30 minutes

1 tablespoon olive oil

1 medium yellow or white onion, coarsely chopped

½ teaspoon salt

2 cloves garlic, minced

1 pound (450 g) chicken breast, cut into 1½" cubes

3 russet potatoes, peeled and cut into large cubes

1 pound (450 g) carrots, cleaned and cut into 1" pieces

3 cans (14½ ounces each) (400 ml each) low-sodium vegetable broth

1 can (14½ ounces) (400 g) whole green beans, with liquid

½ cup (120 ml) ketchup

1 box (10 ounces) (280 g) frozen peas

3 tablespoons Worcestershire sauce

1 teaspoon hot paprika

½ teaspoon black pepper

½ teaspoon red-pepper flakes

In an 8-quart stockpot or Dutch oven, heat the oil over medium heat. Add the onion and salt and cook for 5 minutes, or until the onion is translucent.

Add the garlic and cook for 4 minutes, or until golden. Add the chicken and cook for 10 minutes, or until no longer pink.

Add the potatoes, carrots, broth, green beans, and ketchup. Cook until the stew boils, stirring occasionally.

Reduce the heat to low and add the peas, Worcestershire sauce, paprika, black pepper, and red-pepper flakes. Cook for 1 hour, or until the potatoes and carrots are tender.

Makes 8 servings

PER SERVING: 260 calories, 19 g protein, 34 g carbohydrates, 6 g fat, 33 mg cholesterol, 945 mg sodium, 7 g fiber

Pasta with Shellfish and Mushrooms 480 Calories

Prep time: 10 minutes; Cook time: 15 minutes

1 tablespoon olive oil

1 tin (10 ounces) (280 g) baby clams, with juice

1 pound (450 g) shrimp, peeled and deveined

2 cups (140 g) sliced mushrooms

2 large tomatoes, peeled and coarsely chopped

2 cloves garlic, minced

1 tablespoon fresh dillweed or 1 teaspoon dried dillweed

Salt

Ground black pepper

8 ounces (230 g) whole wheat linguine

⅓ cup (40 g) grated Parmesan cheese

Warm the oil in a large saucepan over medium-high heat. When it's hot, add the clams, shrimp, and mushrooms. Cook, stirring occasionally, for about 5 minutes, or until the shrimp are pink and the mushrooms are soft. Add the tomatoes, garlic, and dillweed. Reduce the heat to low and simmer for about 10 minutes, or until the juice from the tomatoes evaporates a bit. Season to taste with the salt and pepper.

Meanwhile, in a large pot, cook the linguine according to package directions. Drain the pasta and place it in a large bowl. Add the shellfish mixture and toss gently to combine. Sprinkle with the cheese and additional dillweed, if using, and serve.

Makes 4 servings

PER SERVING: 480 calories, 46 g protein, 51 g carbohydrates, 11 g fat, 235 mg cholesterol, 645 mg sodium, 3 g fiber

Kitchen Tip

If you blanch your tomatoes, their skins will slip off easily. Core the tomatoes, removing the stems and white middles. Then cut an X in the bottom of each tomato, cutting only the skin. Bring a pot of water to a boil and add the tomatoes to the water. Boil for about 30 seconds. Remove the tomatoes from the pot and immediately plunge them into ice water to stop the cooking process. When the tomatoes are cool enough to handle, use the edge of the knife to slip off the skin.

Salmon with White Beans and Watercress 286 Calories

Prep time: 10 minutes; Cook time: 15 minutes

4 salmon fillets (4 ounces/140 g each)

Salt and black pepper

2 tablespoons water

2 cloves garlic, minced

1 can (14–19 ounces) (450 g) cannellini beans, rinsed and drained

4 plum tomatoes, chopped

½ cup (120 ml) fat-free chicken broth

1 bunch watercress, rinsed and coarsely chopped

¼ cup (4 tablespoons) chopped Italian parsley

Coat a broiler-pan rack with cooking spray. Preheat the broiler.

Season the fillets with salt and pepper and place on the prepared rack. Broil 4" from the heat for 3 minutes per side, or until just opaque.

Meanwhile, bring the water to a boil in a large nonstick skillet over medium-high heat. Add the garlic and stir for 1 minute. Add the beans, tomatoes, and broth and cook, stirring occasionally, for 3 minutes, or until heated through. Add the watercress and parsley and cook for 30 seconds, or until the watercress begins to wilt. Season with salt and pepper. Serve with the salmon.

Makes 4 servings

PER SERVING: 286 calories, 29 g protein, 17 g carbohydrates, 13 g fat, 65 mg cholesterol, 410 mg sodium, 5 g fiber

Healthy and Delicious Spinach Lasagna 310 Calories

Prep time: 20 minutes; Bake time: 1 hour, 15 minutes

2 cups (480 g) fat-free ricotta cheese

1 package (10 ounces) (300 g) frozen chopped spinach, thawed and squeezed dry

1 egg or ¼ cup (60ml) egg substitute

1 teaspoon dried basil

½ teaspoon Italian seasoning

½ teaspoon salt

¼ teaspoon black pepper

2 cups (8 ounces) (240 g) part-skim mozzarella cheese

1 jar (28 ounces) (800 g) spaghetti sauce

6 whole wheat lasagna noodles

1 cup (240 ml) water

Preheat the oven to 350°F (180°C).

In a medium bowl, combine the ricotta, spinach, egg or egg substitute, basil, Italian seasoning, salt, pepper, and 1 cup (120 g) of the mozzarella.

Evenly spread one-third of the spaghetti sauce in a 13" × 9" baking dish. Top with 3 lasagna noodles. Spread half of the cheese mixture over the noodles. Repeat. Top with the remaining sauce and the remaining 1 cup (120 g) mozzarella. Add the water around the corners of the baking dish. Cover tightly with foil.

Bake for 1 hour and 15 minutes, or until hot and bubbly.

Makes 8 servings

PER SERVING: 310 calories, 19 g protein, 27 g carbohydrates, 15 g fat, 59 mg cholesterol, 913 mg sodium, 3 g fiber

Rolled Swiss Chicken 201 Calories

Prep time: 15 minutes; Cook time: 20 minutes

4 boneless, skinless chicken breast halves (450 g), pounded to ¼" thickness

2 thin slices (about 2 ounces) (60 g) reduced-fat Swiss cheese, cut in half

2 roasted red pepper strips, halved (optional)

8 leaves fresh basil (optional)

2 tablespoons unbleached or all-purpose flour

½ teaspoon ground black pepper

1 tablespoon olive oil

¾ cup (180 ml) reduced-sodium chicken broth

¼ teaspoon dried oregano

Place the chicken on a work surface. Top each piece with half a slice of the cheese, a pepper strip (if using), and 2 basil leaves (if using). Starting from the short ends, tightly roll up the chicken. Tie securely with kitchen string or secure with a wooden pick.

On waxed paper, combine the flour and black pepper. Dredge the chicken rolls in the flour mixture to coat.

Heat the oil in a large nonstick skillet over medium heat. Add the chicken rolls and cook, turning frequently, for 5 minutes, or until golden. Add the broth and oregano and bring to a boil over medium-high heat. Reduce the heat to low and simmer for 15 minutes, or until a thermometer inserted in the thickest portion registers 160°F and the juices run clear. The sauce should be slightly thickened. Remove and discard the string or wooden picks before serving.

Makes 4 servings

PER SERVING: 201 calories, 31 g protein, 4 g carbohydrates, 6 g fat, 71 mg cholesterol, 131 mg sodium, 0 g fiber

Shrimp and Feta Spinach Fettuccine 440 Calories

Prep time: 10 minutes; Cook time: 8 minutes

16 ounces (450 g) spinach fettuccine

1 pound (450 g) frozen cooked shrimp

¼ cup (60 ml) white wine

1 jar (6 ounces) (170 g) marinated artichoke hearts

4 ounces (120 g) oil-packed sun-dried tomatoes, sliced

½ cup (2 ounces) (60 g) tomato-basil feta cheese

3 tablespoons grated Parmesan cheese

½ teaspoon garlic powder or garlic salt

Prepare the pasta according to package directions. Place the shrimp in a strainer under cool running water to thaw. When the pasta is done, pour it into the strainer with the shrimp. Rinse with hot water and drain. Add the wine, tossing to coat as the wine drains.

In a large bowl, combine the artichoke hearts, tomatoes, and feta. Add the pasta mixture to the artichoke mixture and toss to combine. Sprinkle with the Parmesan and season with the garlic powder or garlic salt.

Makes 6 servings

PER SERVING: 440 calories, 31 g protein, 61 g carbohydrates, 9 g fat, 153 mg cholesterol, 515 mg sodium, 5 g fiber

Marinated Grilled Salmon 180 Calories

Prep time: 5 minutes; Marinate time: 1 hour, 30 minutes; Cook time: 10 minutes

¼ cup plus 2 tablespoons (60 ml plus 30 ml) low-sodium soy sauce

¼ cup plus 2 tablespoons (60 ml plus 30 ml) white Zinfandel wine

1 pound (450 g) salmon steaks

1 teaspoon salt-free garlic and herb seasoning divided

In a shallow pan, combine the soy sauce and wine. Add the salmon and turn to coat both sides. Coat the top of the salmon with half of the garlic and herb seasoning. Cover and refrigerate for 45 minutes. Turn the salmon and coat the top with the rest of the seasoning. Cover and refrigerate for 45 minutes longer.

Coat a grill rack with cooking spray. Preheat the grill.

Turn the fish in the marinade, recoating both sides. Place on the grill and cook for 10 minutes, or until the fish flakes easily. Discard the marinade.

Makes 4 servings

PER SERVING: 180 calories, 23 g protein, 1 g carbohydrate, 7 g fat, 62 mg cholesterol, 664 mg sodium, 0 g fiber

Asparagus Medley 90 Calories

Prep time: 10 minutes; Cook time: 8 minutes

1 pound (450 g) asparagus, ends trimmed and stems cut into bite-size pieces

8 ripe olives, sliced

2 plum tomatoes, finely chopped

½ red onion, finely chopped

1 clove garlic, minced

1 tablespoon olive oil

2 tablespoons crumbled feta cheese

Preheat the broiler.

Combine the asparagus, olives, tomatoes, onion, and garlic in a jelly-roll pan. Drizzle with the oil and toss to coat. Sprinkle with the cheese and broil for 8 minutes, or until lightly browned and crisp-tender.

Makes 4 servings

PER SERVING: 90 calories, 3 g protein, 8 g carbohydrates, 5 g fat, 5 mg cholesterol, 130 mg sodium, 3 g fiber

Grilled Eggplant 21 Calories

Prep time: 5 minutes; Marinate time: 1 hour; Cook time: 7 minutes

1 medium eggplant (450 g)
⅓ cup (80 g) fat-free Italian dressing

Cut the eggplant into ½" slices and place in a shallow dish. Pour the dressing over the eggplant and marinate for up to 1 hour, turning occasionally to allow the dressing to completely cover the slices.

Coat a grill rack with cooking spray. Preheat the grill.

Remove the eggplant from the marinade and place on the grill rack. Cook for 7 minutes, turning once, or until slightly charred and tender. Discard the marinade.

Makes 4 servings

PER SERVING: 21 calories, 1 g protein, 5 g carbohydrates, 0 g fat, 0 mg cholesterol, 180 mg sodium, 1 g fiber

Sautéed Yellow Squash, Zucchini, and Onions 149 Calories

Prep time: 5 minutes; Cook time: 15 minutes

2 tablespoons olive oil

2 onions, cut into ¼" slices

2 zucchini, cut in half lengthwise, then cut into ¼" slices

2 yellow squash, cut in half lengthwise, then cut into ¼" slices

3 cloves garlic, finely chopped

½ cup (120 ml) white wine

Salt

Ground black pepper

¼ teaspoon Italian seasoning

Place the oil in a large saucepan over medium-high heat. Add the onions and cook for 3 to 5 minutes, or until translucent. Add the zucchini and the yellow squash and cook for 4 to 5 minutes, stirring occasionally. Add the garlic and cook for 30 seconds. Add the wine, salt and pepper to taste, and Italian seasoning. Cook for 2 to 3 minutes, or until the liquid has reduced by half.

Makes 4 servings

PER SERVING: 149 calories, 3 g protein, 15 g carbohydrates, 7 g fat, 0 mg cholesterol, 14 mg sodium, 5 g fiber

Index

Boldface page references indicate photographs.

Underscored references indicate boxed text.

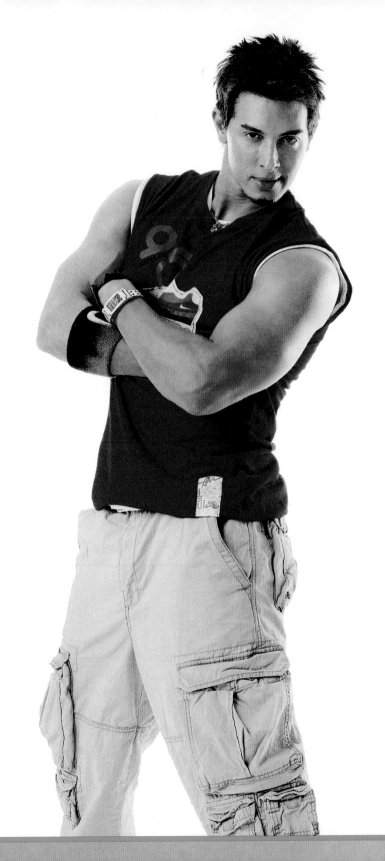

About the Author

One of today's hottest directors and choreographers, Jamie King is continually sought after to work with top stars like Jennifer Lopez, Christina Aguilera, Prince, Ellen Degeneres, Shakira, Rihanna, Mariah Carey, Ricky Martin, Michael Jackson, George Michael, Diana Ross, Elton John, and most notably, his longtime collaborator, Madonna. Most recently, Jamie King directed Madonna's hit music video "Sorry" and directed her record-breaking 2006 *Confessions* world tour. In 2006, Variety named Jamie King as one of the most influential people in the music industry, branding him as "the Jerry Bruckheimer of tentpole concert tours."

In addition to Madonna's *Confessions* tour, in 2006 to 2007, King also directed Christina Aguilera's *Back to Basics* world tour, Ricky Martin's *Black and White* world tour, and Asian superstar Rain's world tour. He previously directed Madonna's *Drowned World* world tour as well as her *Re-Invention* world tour (the highest-grossing tour of 2004), in addition to Pink's *Try This,* Christina Aguilera's *Stripped,* Britney Spears *Oops, I Did It Again,* and Ricky Martin's *La Vida Loca* world tours. Notably, Jamie King created and choreographed Ricky Martin's breakout show-stopping performance of "The Cup of Life" at the 1999 Grammy Awards.

King has collaborated with some of the biggest names in show business, including John Baptiste Mondino, Matthew Rolston, Kenny Ortega, Benny Medina, Steven Klein, David Lachapelle, Wayne Isham, and Quincy Jones.

The creator of the live stage show "Storm" at Las Vegas resort Mandalay Bay, King also choreographed "Tarzan Live" for Disney World's Animal Kingdom, hosted the MTV series "The Grind," and appeared as a celebrity judge on Fox Network's reality series "Dance Fever."

Not only is Jamie King known for his work with celebrities, he's also been creating quite a sensation as the creator of the Nike Rockstar Workout, which has become hugely popular at health clubs across the country and around the world. King is Nike's creative consultant and global spokesperson for the Nike dance fitness product line.

Jamie King has been nominated for three Emmy Awards (Prince tribute on the American Music Awards; Madonna's *Drowned World* Tour HBO special; and the 68th Annual Academy Awards) and has been nominated for five MTV Music Video Awards ("I'm Glad"—Jennifer Lopez; "Die Another Day"—Madonna; "Don't Tell Me"—Madonna; "Human Nature"—Madonna; and "Hung Up"—Madonna). He lives in Beverly Hills, California.

www.jamiekingofficial.com